Informed Consent for
Blood Transfusion

Informed Consent for Blood Transfusion

Editor

Christopher P. Stowell, MD, PhD
Director, Blood Transfusion Service
Massachusetts General Hospital
Department of Pathology
Harvard Medical School
Boston, Massachusetts

American Association of Blood Banks
Bethesda, Maryland
1997

American Association of Blood Banks
8101 Glenbrook Road
Bethesda, Maryland 20814-2749

ISBN 1-56395-087-1
Printed in the United States

Contents

A Letter from the President

Dear Colleague:

On behalf of the membership of the American Association of Blood Banks (AABB), I am pleased to present this updated resource on informed consent. After much research and revision, this long awaited work is now available to assist health-care providers as they develop innovative policies and procedures to meet informed consent requirements for blood transfusion.

The AABB has recommended disclosing the risks and benefits of transfusion therapy to patients facing transfusion decisions since Past President Eugene M. Berkman, MD issued his July 10, 1986 memorandum to all AABB institutional members. In February 1989, the AABB sponsored a conference on this topic and published the proceedings. Later that year, the association published *Informed Consent for Blood Transfusion—A Physician's Resource Kit.*

The medical and legal fields rapidly evolved over the ensuing years and by September 1994 it was apparent that the resource kit had become outdated. To address this problem, AABB Past President Charles Wallas, MD, issued AABB Association Bulletin #94-3 revising and reaffirming the Association's position on informed consent for blood transfusion. He also assigned the AABB's Scientific Section Coordinating Committee the task of updating and expanding the AABB resources on informed consent. This publication is the result of that process.

The title of the work, *Informed Consent for Blood Transfusion*, reflects the increasing acceptance that the duty to provide informed consent for blood transfusion transcends the treating physicians and may extend to hospitals and other health-care providers. This view is reflected in the Joint Commission on Accreditation of Healthcare Organization requirement that hospitals obtain informed consent for blood transfusion before surgery in which there is a "possibility" that blood will be transfused.

Other key benefits of this book include a more detailed discussion of the risks, benefits, and alternatives to transfusion. In addition, the chapter on developing and implementing informed consent policies and procedures in the hospital setting has been considerably expanded and is much more explicit than in previous publications.

This publication answers a need that has been strongly expressed by medical professionals for some time. While the suggestions included in this publication are not official AABB policy and should not be construed as AABB standards, the association offers this publication as a resource for institutions as they develop and refine their policies and procedures for providing informed consent for blood transfusion.

Sincerely,
Dennis M. Smith, Jr., MD
1996-97 AABB President

Foreword

Since the initial AABB publications on informed consent were offered, the application of the informed consent process to the transfusion of blood and its derivatives has become widely accepted and practiced. Indeed, some states have adopted statutory requirements in this area. However, some institutions are still wrestling with the development and implementation of an informed consent policy. Many are attempting to adapt their policies to the evolving concept of informed consent in health care in general, as well as in its specific application to transfusion.

Recognizing the continued need for guidance and the changes in our concept of informed consent, the AABB offers this up-to-date resource. It is important to note that, because of the significant changes that have occurred since 1989 in both the practice of transfusion medicine and in the law, the earlier publications should be regarded as outdated.

The scope of the book has been broadened to include information on informed consent that is applicable to physicians *and* hospitals. Although the duty to inform still lies with the physician, recent case law should serve as a warning to hospitals that they may be responsible for implementing procedures to provide informed consent.

K. Sazama, MD, JD reviews the legal basis for informed consent and its development. A summary of key litigation that has molded our concepts of informed consent in the transfusion setting is provided by P. Schiff, JD and J.P. Barber, JD of the AABB counsel's office. At the core of the informed consent process is the discussion of the risks, benefits, and alternatives to transfusion. These discussions, which a patient requires to make an informed decision, are covered in a series of four chapters by Drs. Chambers, Kleinman, and Stowell.

Finally, Drs. Lane, Sniecinski and Stowell review key issues that must be addressed in the process of establishing an informed consent policy for an institution. Sample procedures and forms are provided for illustration. The AABB does not specifically endorse the use of any of these materials; rather, they are presented as examples of how an institution may deal with the issues of conveying information to patients and documenting the process of informed consent.

Physicians and other health-care workers dealing directly with transfusion recipients or persons developing educational programs for these professionals may find the chapters on the risks, benefits, and alternatives to allogeneic transfusion of greatest use. Those who are developing or reviewing institutional policies on informed consent will find the chapters on the legal background and procedure development the most helpful.

State and local laws govern the legal requirements of informed consent for transfusion and should be reviewed carefully. This publication does not purport to identify or discuss the nuances of the many different state (and possibly local) requirements regarding informed consent. In addition, the constantly-shifting legal and legislative environment make periodic review of existing informed consent policies imperative. Although every effort has been made to provide the most current published information on the risks, benefits, and alternatives to transfusion, this area of medicine is changing rapidly. In particular, risk estimates for transfusion complications are subject to revision as methods for reducing or avoiding them are implemented and as new hazards are appreciated.

Informed Consent for Blood Transfusions is offered by the Scientific Section Coordinating Committee of the AABB as a resource to help hospitals, physicians, and others dealing with the policy and practice of informed consent for blood transfusion.

Christopher Stowell, MD, PhD
Editor

In: Stowell, CP, ed.
Informed Consent for Blood Transfusion
Bethesda, MD: American Association of Blood Banks, 1997

1

Informed Consent for Transfusion: An Overview

Kathleen Sazama, MD, JD

The doctrine of informed consent has assumed increasing importance during the 15 years since the first occurrence of transfusion-transmitted human immunodeficiency virus (HIV), the virus that causes acquired immune deficiency syndrome (AIDS). More than 800 lawsuits have been filed as a result of transfusion-transmitted HIV.[1] A number of these cases include claims for negligent nondisclosure of risks associated with transfusion (ie, lack of informed consent). Decisions in these cases continue to refine the doctrine of informed consent as applied to transfusion medicine.[2] Although most hospitals currently require written informed consent for nonemergency-related transfusion, the practice in most institutions generally fails to meet the legal requirements.[3] Perhaps in recognition of the need to address this increasingly important aspect of patient care, in 1995 the Joint Commission on Accreditation of Healthcare Organizations added the requirement for informed consent for blood transfusion to its standards for hospital accreditation.[4] All hospitals that transfuse blood and blood components and every physician who may order transfusions should have a clear understanding of, and operational poli-

Kathleen Sazama, MD, JD, Professor of Pathology and Laboratory Medicine, Medical College of Pennsylvania and Hahnemann University, Philadelphia, Pennsylvania

cies and procedures in place for, obtaining informed consent from patients whose care includes transfusion therapy.

The Origins of Informed Consent

The Law

The law has long protected persons from unwanted touching (battery) or fear of being touched (assault).[5] These principles were first articulated in the context of medicine in an 18th century English court decision *Slater v. Baker & Stapleton,*[6] which held that two medical practitioners should not have separated the ends of a healing fracture without the consent of the patient. For the next century, courts developed assault and battery theories to provide recovery in cases involving patients who were injured as a result of medical procedures for which they had not provided consent.

In 1905 one court summarized the US law up to that point as follows: "Under a free government at least, the free citizen's first and greatest right which underlies all others—the right to the inviolability of his person, in other words, his right to himself, is the subject of universal acquiescence and this right necessarily forbids a physician . . . to violate without permission the bodily integrity of his patient by a major or capital operation."[7] The protection of the law was then extended in the 1914 decision in *Schloendorff v. Society of New York Hospital,* in which Justice Cardozo articulated the right of self-determination to include choices beyond those involving surgery in the statement, "Every human being of adult years and sound mind has a right to determine what shall be done with his own body . . . ."[8] The *Schloendorff* decision is frequently cited as the origin of the doctrine of consent in US law. Taken together, these cases provided considerable protection for individual autonomy, ensuring that patients could recover for medical assault or battery if they could show that they did not consent, expressly or through implication, to the medical treatment received.

The early common law, however, failed to provide recovery in situations in which patients consented to procedures that caused them injury, but the consent was based on inadequate information. To provide a remedy for these patients, courts began applying negligence theories to allow recovery for cases in which physicians failed to properly disclose all information about the risks of the proposed procedure. Generally, under negligence theories it has been the physicians who owe their patients a duty to disclose all material risks of a proposed procedure prior to obtaining consent for the procedure. In fact, patients are entitled to recovery if the physician's disclosure falls short of this standard and as a result they consented to a procedure that caused injury. However, it is important that hospital administrators also recognize the significance of making sure that informed consent policies are provided. Legal theories of corporate negligence and respondeat superior have been applied in some cases to assess liability for instituting good informed consent programs. Chapter 2 includes a more detailed analysis of the application of negligence theories in informed consent cases.

Informed consent is a process that depends upon adequate communication between a competent patient and the physician who will provide the care under discussion.[9] In his inauguration speech, American Medical Association President Daniel H. Johnson, MD, said that "under the doctrine of informed consent the physician cannot make a decision for a patient, but must instead serve as a counselor to the patient." The basic requirements to be communicated in informed consent discussions are identified in Table 1-1. Foremost among these requirements is the affirmative obligation of disclosure of information by the physician to the patient. The physician is responsible for educating each patient about the specific proposed course of treatment so that the patient can intelligently share in responsible decision-making. Implicit in this principle is the right of a patient to decline the proposed treatment or procedure.

Ethics

The right of informed consent derives from the ethics of our society as well as from the law. In 1982 a presidential commission

Table 1-1. Elements of Informed Consent

Information Provided by Physician

- Risks of treatment
- Benefits of treatment
- Alternative treatments

Opportunity for Questions and Clarification

- Patient competency
- Patient (or surrogate decision maker) understands
- Patient decides on basis of complete information

Patient Agrees or Refuses

Documentation

---

issued a comprehensive report assessing patient rights in medical and investigational research settings. This report is viewed as a cornerstone of the modern ethics of informed consent.[10] It states that in ethics, principles of individual autonomy, self-determination, beneficence, nonmaleficence, and justice underlie patient rights. The key concepts for ethicists in informed consent for treatment include disclosure, comprehension, voluntariness, competence, and consent. An act is presumed to be informed consent "if a patient . . . agrees to an intervention based on an understanding of relevant information, the consent is not controlled by influences that engineer the outcome, and the consent given was intended to be a consent and therefore qualified as a permission for an intervention."[11] The AMA, numerous state medical societies, and other medical professional organizations have incorporated the ethical principles of informed consent into modern practice.

The Doctrine of Informed Consent

Necessary Elements

Before any treatment or procedure occurs, patients have the right to decide whether they wish to receive the treatment or procedure. Patients decide on the basis of their understanding of why the recommendation is being made, what risks and benefits accompany the circumstance, whether any alternatives to the proposal realistically exist, and any other concerns that they may have. To ensure that patients have the information they need to make an informed choice, the physician should provide it in language the patient understands.[12] The information should include, as a minimum, the following (taken from Annas' *The Rights of Patients*)[9]:

1. A description of the *recommended treatment* or procedure.
2. A description of the *risks and benefits* of the recommended procedure, with special emphasis on the risks of death or serious bodily disability.
3. A description of the *alternatives*, including other treatments or procedures together with the risks and benefits of these alternatives.
4. The likely results of *no treatment*.
5. The *probability of success*, and what the physician means by success.
6. The major problems anticipated in *recuperation*, and the length of time during which the patient will not be able to resume his or her normal activities.
7. Any other information generally provided to patients in this situation by other qualified physicians.

Again, underlying all legal and ethical requirements for informed consent is the individual patient's right to refuse. Refusal of consent requires no different documentation than agreement. Only in the context of a surrogate decision-maker or with issues of competency would a challenge to refusal exist. Because it is the patient's choice, the right to refuse must be honored. Otherwise, the right of informed consent would deteriorate into little more than the requirement to agree with the physician.

Disclosure: What, How, to Whom

Foremost in patient concern, as evidenced by court decisions, is to what risks the patient will be subjected in the proposed course of treatment. Closely allied is whether the patient received the intended benefit. Obviously, alternatives to the actual treatment, when reasonable, frequently provide the impetus to litigate undesirable outcomes.

Risks and Benefits

Patients must be informed of the risks and benefits of recommended diagnostic procedures and treatments, the reasonable alternatives, and the risks and benefits of not performing the treatment or procedure. (See Table 1-2.) Physicians must disclose, at a minimum, any risk of death, significant risks of harm, peculiar risks due to the specific treatment, and risks due to a patient's particular history or condition. Physicians should be particularly careful to disclose the additional risks when discussing any treatment that is:

- Investigational or novel
- Newly approved
- Particularly hazardous
- Capable of altering sexual capacity or fertility
- Purely cosmetic

In circumstances in which the standard of practice is not well-established, such as occurred in the early AIDS era, physicians may want to tell patients that opinions differ among physicians or that there is a great deal of uncertainty or lack of data about the possible outcomes of the proposed treatment. For informed consent to withstand legal scrutiny, physicians in doubt should err on the side of overdisclosure.

When providing medical information to their patients, physicians often use words most intelligible to persons having more than a high school level of education. However, if a physician does not deliberately "translate" scientific and medical terminology, the patient can easily demonstrate that no information exchange occurred. When such a miscommunication relates to risks, particularly significant risks of considerable harm, the physician will likely be held accountable. For transfusion risks, data are regularly updated, generally showing diminishing risks as scientific

Table 1-2. Risks That Should be Disclosed in Informed Consent Discussions With Patients

Primary risks

- Any risk of death
- Significant risks of harm
- Peculiar risks of the specific treatment
- Risks due to a patient's own history or condition

Additional risks related to treatment that is

- Investigational or novel
- Newly approved
- Particularly hazardous
- Capable of altering sexual capacity or fertility
- Purely cosmetic

When the standard of practice is not well-established, discuss

- Differences in opinions
- Uncertainty
- Lack of data

knowledge advances. Information about risk from transfusion as of 1995 is included in Chapters 3 and 4.

Process

A practical approach to disclosure is for hospitals to encourage development of a standard process for physicians to inform patients, targeted to the particular treatment choice, eg, transfusion. The extent to which practicing physicians are informed about transfusion practices is a continuing concern,[13,14] requiring personal effort by the physician as well as reliance on experts in blood banking and transfusion medicine. Some medical school curricula[15] have incorporated, as a priority, education about transfusion medicine,[16] with some measurable success. If hospitals are aware of the need for a standard process and support a program for physicians to use, it should protect both in the event of litigation. Having a written process provides objective evidence that the physician is teaching each patient what is needed to make a decision affecting his or her medical welfare.

The written process can be an outline or information sheet for the patient that includes such topics as what is wrong, what approaches to treatment (including transfusion) are available, what are the benefits and risks (pros and cons) of treatment (specifically the known and current risks of transfusion), what alternatives (pharmacologic, donor source, etc) are realistically available, and what will happen if the patient decides to refuse transfusion. If the treating physician uses the information sheet or outline as a checklist, then the documentation of information-sharing is easy if an issue arises later in the context of a legal matter. However, it is not sufficient to simply hand the patient a written sheet of information and assume that the patient will either read or understand it. The process requires a discussion between patients and physicians in which patients are given ample opportunity to discuss and resolve any questions, issues, or concerns that they may have relative to the proposed transfusion before they agree to (or refuse) it.

The time spent discussing the intended intervention may be an important element. If the physician creates an atmosphere that could be interpreted as coercive because insufficient time or attention is devoted to the patient's concerns, even the best planned process will not insulate the physician from liability.

The documentation frequently consumes much time and energy but is, at best, only evidence of the preceding discussion and consent. Obviously, documentation assumes greater importance in the context of refusal for transfusion, especially when such refusals are due to religious objections.[17] Some examples of documentation for the informed consent process are included in Chapter 7.

Withdrawal of Consent

Consent can be withdrawn *at any time.* As a practical matter, no patient who is under anesthesia or other medication that alters consciousness, who is comatose, or who is in significant pain can withdraw consent previously given. However, once a patient has identified an intention to revoke or withdraw previous consent, the physician must accept the withdrawal at once.

Conclusion

During the past decade, the public has become increasingly knowledgeable about risks of transfusion, particularly the risk of contracting HIV from transfusion. As a result, physicians—and in a few cases, hospitals—are being targeted in lawsuits for inadequate informed consent in the transfusion setting.[18] The information in the following chapters is intended to offer guidance to those organizations and individuals who may have a requirement to obtain informed consent, including practicing clinicians and hospitals.

References

1. Shepherd LL. The risk of transfusion-associated AIDS: Offering patients an active role in their care. Am J Med Qual 1992;7:111-15.
2. Bierig JR. Legal issues for blood banks. Arch Pathol Lab Med 1994;118:442-53.
3. Eisenstaedt RS, Glanz K, Smith DG, Derstine T. Informed consent for blood transfusion: A regional hospital survey. Transfusion 1993;33:558-61.
4. Comprehensive accreditation manual for hospitals. Oakbrook Terrace, IL: Joint Commission on Accreditation of Healthcare Organizations, 1995.
5. Prosser WL, ed. Law of torts. 4th ed. Denver: Westlaw Publishing Co, 1971, §10.
6. *Slater v. Baker & Stapleton,* 95 Eng. Rep. 860 (K.B. 1767) as cited in Appelbaum PS, Lidz CW, Meisel A. Informed consent. Legal theory and clinical practice. New York: Oxford University Press, 1987:36-7.

7. *Pratt v. Davis,* 118 Ill. App. 161, 166 (1905), *aff'd,* 244 Ill. 30, 79 N.E. 562 (1906).

8. *Schloendorff v. Society of New York Hospital,* 211 N.Y. 125, 105 N.E. 92 (1914).

9. Annas GJ. The rights of patients: The basic ACLU guide to patient rights. Revised edition. Totowa, NJ: Humana Press, 1992.

10. President's Commission for the Study of Ethical Problems in Medicine and Biochemical and Behavioral Research. Making health care decisions: The ethical and legal implications of informed consent in the patient-practitioner relationship. Vol. e, Appendices. Washington, DC: US Government Printing Office,1982.

11. Beauchamp TL. Informed consent. In: Veatch RM, ed. Medical ethics. Boston: Jones and Bartlett Publishers, 1989:174.

12. *Natanson v. Kline,* 350 P.2d 1093 (Kan 1960), *reh'g denied,* 187 Kan 186, 354 P.2d 670 (1960).

13. Crosby ET. Perioperative haemotherapy: II. Risks and complications of blood transfusion. Can J Anaesth 1992;39:822-37.

14. Capen K. Informed consent and blood transfusion: What does Krever's interim report mean to doctors? Can Med Assoc J 1995;152:1663-5.

15. Goodnough LT, Hull AL, Kleinhenz ME. Teaching medical students concepts of informed consent within the framework of a transfusion medicine curriculum. Acad Med 1992;67: 348.

16. Goodnough LT, Hull AL, Kleinhenz ME. Informed consent for blood transfusion as a transfusion medicine educational intervention. Transfus Med 1994;4:51-5.

17. Goldman EB, Oberman HA. Legal aspects of transfusion of Jehovah's Witnesses. Transfus Med Rev 1991;5:263-70.

18. See, eg, *Reyes, et al v. United States,* No. 91-1859 (1st Cir. Jan. 14, 1992); *Hoemke v. New York Blood Center,* No. 90-7182 (2d Cir. Aug. 24, 1990); *Kozup v. Georgetown University,* et al, No. 86-0033 (D.D.C. April 21, 1989) aff'd in part, No. 89-7124 and 7125 (D.C.Cir. July 3, 1990), on remand from 663 F. Supp. 1048 (D.D.C. 1987), aff'd in part, 851 F.2d 437 (D.C.Cir. 1988).

In: Stowell, CP, ed.
Informed Consent for Blood Transfusion
Bethesda, MD: American Association of Blood Banks, 1997

2

Statement of the Law on Informed Consent for Transfusion

Philip D. Schiff, JD, and John Paul Barber, JD

This chapter reviews the legal issues associated with the duties of a health-care provider to fully inform and obtain consent from patients before transfusion of blood and blood components. Before these issues are examined in depth, however, it is important to understand that under our legal system the laws governing informed consent—as well as other theories of legal liability—vary from one state to another throughout the United States.[1]

Federal Regulations

Federal law is silent on the issue of informed consent, with the exception of federal regulations governing the provision of informed consent for patients participating in certain research protocols.[2] These regulations require an institution preparing a medical research protocol to objectively review the proposed treatment before institution of investigational or experimental procedures. This review must include approval of the proposed informed consent process.

Philip D. Schiff, JD, General Counsel and John Paul Barber, JD, Associate General Counsel and Director of Legislative Affairs, American Association of Blood Banks, Bethesda, Maryland

On November 1, 1996, the FDA issued a final rule governing clinical research in medical emergencies. The rule allows health-care providers to test experimental therapies for life-threatening emergencies without a patient's consent, provided that an institutional review board has determined that the therapy would benefit patients and that the community is informed. The rule is being applied in a clinical trial of a blood substitute.[3]

State Laws

Through statutes, regulations, case law, and deliberations of administrative boards, states have defined the legal duty of health-care providers generally to provide patients with the information that they need to make rational choices about their health care. Some states have specific laws that delineate what information must be disclosed for specific diagnoses or conditions. All physicians must become familiar with the peculiarities of state law that apply to their practice and incorporate this information appropriately into their interactions with patients. The nuances of testing for and disclosure of human immunodeficiency virus (HIV) are particularly troublesome because each state has established its own approach.

California, New Jersey, and Pennsylvania have enacted special statutes establishing specific requirements that physicians obtain informed consent from patients who are planning to undergo a medical procedure involving a potential blood transfusion (see Appendices 2-1, 2-2, and 2-3).[4-6] The statutes dictate the specific risks and alternatives (including use of autologous and directed donations) that must be disclosed. Although applicable only in their respective states, the statutes offer a basis for identifying relevant material to be disclosed in the context of providing blood transfusions. Those practicing outside of California, New Jersey, and Pennsylvania may use these statutes as guidelines in the context of developing informed consent procedures for their own facilities.

Other states apply rules developed in medical malpractice cases to analyze transfusion-related informed consent issues.

These rules vary in some respects. As a result, facts that establish legal liability in one jurisdiction may not give rise to such liability in another. Thus, the principles and materials referenced in this chapter should not be viewed as definitive statements of the law throughout the United States. They are only provided as an explanation of the general concepts. Health-care providers offering transfusions to patients should consult with individuals experienced in the local law concerning informed consent before developing and instituting standard operating procedures for providing informed consent to patients for blood transfusion.

General Legal Concepts

Generally, the law of informed consent can be stated as follows:
    In the absence of emergency or unanticipated conditions, a physician or surgeon must first obtain a patient's consent before treating or operating on the patient. However, the patient must be competent to give consent, or someone legally authorized to give consent must agree to the procedure. Additionally, the consent must be given with adequate knowledge of the risks, or it is not valid.[7]
While the core idea of informed consent is relatively straightforward and easy to understand, there are many nuances of this legal theory that must be explored to understand the disclosure obligations that health-care providers owe to patients preparing for blood transfusion therapy.

Battery

As discussed in Chapter 1, courts generally assess a health-care provider's liability for failure to provide informed consent under two legal theories—battery and negligence. In early common law, claims that a patient had been injured as a result of medical treatment to which the patient did not agree were treated as battery—an act by the defendant that brings about harmful or offensive contact to the plaintiff's person. In the medical context, physicians do not commit battery on their patients if they first obtain consent. Conversely, surgeons who operate without their patients' consent commit battery for which they may be liable in damages. However, in the event of a bona fide medical emergency, the patient's consent is implied. (See Chapter 1 for more information about the historical development of battery theories in medical cases.)

Although most lawsuits involving allegations of failure to provide informed consent are now brought under alternative theories of negligence (discussed below), many plaintiffs still include battery claims in their pleadings. In *Traxler v. Vardy*, the plaintiff argued that her physician had committed battery because, although she had consented to a dilation and curettage procedure, she did not consent to the transfusion that followed the operation. The court recognized that under California law, when a patient gives permission to perform one type of treatment and the physician performs another, a battery is committed. However, the court refused to find that the accompanying blood transfusion was a "second procedure" outside the scope of the patient's original consent.[8(p 304)]

In Pennsylvania the doctrine of informed consent is grounded in battery. As a result, the duty to provide informed consent in that state is limited to cases involving surgical procedures. Since blood transfusion was not considered a surgical procedure per se, in the past it was unclear whether informed consent for blood transfusion was legally required in Pennsylvania. In *Hoffman v. Brandywine Hospital*, a Pennsylvania state court held that the treating physician was not required to disclose transfusion risks and alternatives because the transfusion did not occur during surgery.[9] However, a Pennsylvania federal court reasoned that a physician cannot inform a patient of all material risks of a surgical procedure without also informing the patient of transfusion risks when a blood transfusion is a potential part of the procedure.[10(p 1125)] The issue was recently settled when the state legislature enacted legislation mandating informed consent for blood transfusion.[6]

Texas law prohibits battery claims in informed consent cases. In Texas courts, only a negligence theory can be used in a suit against a physician or health-care provider involving a claim based on failure to disclose or to adequately disclose the risks associated with the medical care or surgical procedure rendered.[11]

Negligence

To succeed in assessing liability against a health-care provider for failure to properly inform under a negligence theory, patients (or their representatives) must show the following[12]:

- The defendant health-care provider owed a duty to the patient to disclose the risk involved in the proposed treatment.
- There was a breach of that duty.
- The breach was the proximate cause of the injury.
- There was in fact a legally compensable injury.

Duty to Provide Informed Consent

Physician's Duty

Prior to examining in detail the legal theories associated with the duty to provide informed consent, it is useful to understand which parties have this legal responsibility and to whom the risks and benefits of blood transfusion should be disclosed. Generally, the treating physician holds the primary responsibility for disclosing all material risks to the patient who will receive the blood transfusion.[13] In some circumstances physicians may delegate this duty to other health-care providers.[14] In many jurisdictions the duty to provide informed consent is broadening to include hospitals as well as other health-care providers. Additionally, in some situations it is appropriate to obtain informed consent from an individual other than the transfusion recipient.

Hospital's Duty

As noted, the obligation to provide informed consent is a duty that physicians owe to their patients.[15] Traditionally, this responsibility has not been shifted to the hospital or any other health-care provider.[16] For example, a Texas court of appeals dismissed informed consent claims against a hospital, noting that the claims followed the physician.[13] A Pennsylvania court dismissed informed consent claims against a cardiologist because he was not the physician who actually performed the surgery.[17] An Oklahoma Court of Appeals reasoned that imposing a duty on hospitals to provide informed consent intervenes in the physician-patient relationship and causes more disruption than benefit to the patient. The Oklahoma court therefore concluded that it is the duty of the physician ordering blood transfusions, rather than the hospital filling the physician's orders, to inform patients of the risks involved in a transfusion.[18] In reaching its decision, the court determined that treating physicians are uniquely qualified—through education and training and as a result of their relationship to the patient—to provide proper informed consent.

It should be recognized, however, that the verdicts against hospitals are increasing. Although a New Mexico appellate court refused to impose a duty to provide informed consent on hospital staff, the court recognized that in some special circumstances a hospital can be held liable for a physician's failure to provide informed consent under the "corporate negligence theory."[19(p 797)] A hospital may be liable for a physician's negligence on the basis of the hospital's "failure to properly oversee the treatment of its patients."[19(p 800)] An Illinois Court of Appeals also applied the corporate negligence doctrine to impose a duty on hospitals to require physicians using their facilities to provide informed consent.[20]

The Supreme Court of Washington ruled on a slightly different basis that a hospital can be liable for the failure of its medical staff to provide informed consent. Applying the concept of "respondeat superior," in which an employer is responsible for the acts of its employees (and no separate negligence by the employer is required), the Washington court reasoned that hospitals have a duty to exercise reasonable care in selecting, retaining, and supervising medical staff.[21]

Additionally, Washington courts have specifically required hospitals to provide informed consent in extraordinary situations in which hospital staff are aware of a risk specific to an individual patient.[21] Even though a hospital may not have an independent legal duty to obtain informed consent, if it gratuitously undertakes the obligation, it has a duty to make certain that the disclosure fully informs patients of the risks associated with blood transfusion.[10(p 1131)]

Hospital liability could be expanded by a new policy established by the Joint Commission on Accreditation of Healthcare Organization (JCAHO), requiring that hospitals have procedures in place for providing informed consent for blood transfusion.[22] If courts construe the JCAHO policy as the standard of care for hospitals, hospitals that do not provide informed consent for blood transfusion could be held liable. It should also be noted that even if a court finds that the hospital owes a duty to provide informed consent, this does not necessarily relieve treating physicians of their duty to their patients.

Duty of Hospitals and Blood Collection Centers to Disseminate Information

Blood collection facilities and hospitals have legal duties to provide information sufficient to enable physicians to communicate effectively with their patients about blood transfusions. The blood collector's duty is to act reasonably in providing accurate information to others under the theory of the "learned intermediary" so that the physicians or transfusers of the blood can discharge their duties to their patients.[23] Such information could include data about transfusion risks and details regarding available alternatives to allogeneic transfusion (see Chapters 3 and 4).

Duty Is Owed to the Patient

The law presumes adult persons to be competent to make decisions regarding medical care.[24] The health-care provider must obtain informed consent from the person who will actually receive the transfusion unless it is clear that the patient is not competent to make that decision. Adult patients with permanent disabilities such as mental illness and overt physical limitations should be accorded the same presumption of competency as any other patient.[25] When mental illness has been diagnosed, assessment of competency should be made by a mental health professional familiar with the patient. Sometimes, because of acute illness or injury, the patient is competent only intermittently or transiently. In such circumstances, careful observation and complete documentation of status changes will establish the reliability of informed consent obtained during lucid intervals. Consent efforts during such intervals should document the same discussion of information as for any other competent person, with a record of what treatment decision was made by the patient and when.

Surrogate Decision-Makers

Consent must be obtained from a surrogate decision-maker if the patient appears to be incompetent, underage (according to state law), comatose, or severely mentally retarded; has profound organic brain syndrome; or has already been judged to be incompetent. The surrogate decision-maker may be a family member, a court-appointed legal guardian, or the court itself.

Legal safeguards exist to protect the patient's rights even when a surrogate decision-maker acts for the patient. When a substituted judgment is made on behalf of an incompetent patient, the surrogate decision-maker should consider the patient's actual interests, preferences, and present and future incompetency. Ultimately, the decision should be the one that the patient would have made if competent.[26] Courts have overruled parental decisions to refuse transfusion on religious grounds when the transfusion was deemed in the best interests of the child.[27]

Minors

Before administering treatment—including transfusion—to minors, physicians must obtain informed consent from a parent or guardian, except in emergency situations in which either the child's life is in danger or a delay may result in significant morbidity. State law determines the age of consent and whether consent by a parent or legal guardian is required for transfusion and other medical assistance. Many states have adopted the concept of "emancipated minors," children who can make decisions for themselves and are not subject to parental control. Emancipation is often based on whether the minor is married, has children, is in military service, or attends college. Courts may also use the "mature minor" standard to evaluate the adequacy of informed consent. Under this standard the court considers the minor's age, ability to understand the proposed treatment, and whether the risks and benefits (particularly when serious risks exist) have been adequately and appropriately explained and understood.[28] There may be additional specific state requirements when the minor is being seen for certain medical conditions, usually including treatment of venereal disease, consequences of intravenous drug or alcohol abuse, and pregnancy. When the minor agrees to receive transfusions or infusions, the adequacy of informed consent will take into account all of these restrictions.

Physician-Oriented View of Duty

When disagreements arise regarding whether consent was informed, the courts have depended on various legal standards to determine whether the physician owed a duty to disclose the risk in question. Traditionally, a physician's duty to provide informed consent has been measured by a *professional standard of care.* Under this analysis, physicians are required to provide information about the risks associated with the proposed medical treatment that physicians consider to be "material." Under this standard, material information is determined by considering the customary disclosure practices of other physicians in the area or what a reasonable physician would disclose under the same or similar circumstances. Thus to prevail on an informed consent claim under this standard, plaintiffs must show, through expert testimony, that other physicians in the area were disclosing the particular risk or that a reasonable physician in the same circumstances would have disclosed the risk.[7]

In *Sawyer v. Methodist Hospital,* the court applied the professional standard of care to dismiss a transfusion-related informed consent claim. The plaintiff alleged that had he known of the risk of transfusion-transmitted hepatitis, he would have refused the blood transfusion. Finding that at the time of the 1972 transfusion, it was not the practice of Memphis-area physicians to warn patients of the possibility of hepatitis transmission before administering a blood transfusion, the district court held that the physician did not owe a duty to disclose the risk of transfusion-transmitted hepatitis.[29(p 1102)]

Patient-Oriented View of Duty

Beginning in California in 1957, the courts began to measure a physician's duty to inform a patient of the risks of a treatment or procedure not by what other professionals disclose, but by the patient's need for information that is *material* to the decision to accept or reject the proposed treatment. If the risks of a proposed procedure are found to be material, the treating physician has a duty to disclose these risks.

In *Salgo v. Leland Stanford Jr. University Board of Trustees*,[30] Salgo, who became paralyzed as a complication of translumbar aortography, asserted that not only was the physician negligent in performing the procedure, he had failed to inform Salgo of the risks, including paralysis. Salgo further claimed that a reasonable person should be informed of the risks before agreeing to undergo the procedure. The court agreed with Salgo, for the first time using the term "informed consent" to require that physicians provide sufficient information to permit an intelligent consent by ensuring full disclosure of facts necessary ("material" in legal terms) to make this decision.

In *Canterbury v. Spence*, one of the leading informed consent cases applying the patient view, the Washington, DC Circuit Court held that in order to prevail with an informed consent claim grounded in negligence, a plaintiff must show the following[31(p 772)]:

- There was a material risk associated with a course of treatment.

- The plaintiff's physician failed to disclose the material risk.
- If the material risk had been disclosed, the plaintiff would have declined that course of treatment.
- The treatment injured the plaintiff.

The *Canterbury* court defined materiality as an objective standard, holding that a risk is material if a reasonable person in the patient's position would be likely to attach significance to the risk in deciding whether to forgo the proposed therapy.[31(p 787)]

Similarly, California juries are routinely instructed that a physician's duty is to disclose all material information that is needed to enable a patient to make an informed decision regarding the proposed operation or treatment. California juries are told that *material information* is defined objectively as information that the physician knows or should know would be regarded as significant by a *reasonable* person in the patient's position when deciding whether to accept or reject a recommended medical procedure.[8(p 303-4)] Texas defines the material risk concept statutorily, providing that physicians must disclose "the risks or hazards that could have influenced a reasonable person in making a decision to give or withhold consent."[11]

A minority of jurisdictions adhere to the view that material information is determined subjectively by considering what the individual plaintiff, as opposed to a "reasonable plaintiff," would have done with the information.[32,33] This differs from the objective standard in taking into account the particular patient, including his or her emotional and physiologic state at the time of consent, the individual medical history and what information that particular patient needed to know to make the specific medical decision.[29(p 1106)]

While health-care providers should not minimize medical risks, courts recognize that it is unrealistic to expect health-care providers to discuss with their patients every potential risk—no matter how remote—of a proposed treatment. Disclosure is required only when the risk is medically known or foreseeable.[34] Too much disclosure could alarm a patient who is already unduly apprehensive and who, as a result, may refuse to undergo surgery for which there is minimal risk.

Material Risk and Transfusion-Transmitted Diseases

Whether a risk is considered material is a function of both frequency and severity. While scientific data pertaining to the risk of transfusion-transmitted infections may guide a court's determination as to whether the transmission risk is material, courts also consider the magnitude of the transfusion risk in question. In Sawyer, for example, the court of appeals concluded that the 0.013% incidence rate in 1972 of transfusion-transmitted hepatitis at the hospital in question was "extremely remote" and ruled that the physician did not owe a duty to inform the patient of this risk and that Sawyer would not have forgone the procedure on the basis of the risk.[29(p 1107)]

In HIV-transmission lawsuits, whether the risk of HIV transmission from blood transfusion is material and therefore required to be disclosed often depends on when the transfusion occurred. In the early 1980s, the risk of transfusion-transmitted HIV infection often was not clear to physicians or patients. Courts have reached conflicting decisions on whether this risk should have been disclosed at that time. In *Kozup v. Georgetown University*, the district court for the District of Columbia noted that in January 1983—the time of the plaintiff's transfusion—there was still no consensus in the medical or blood banking communities that the causative agent for AIDS was transmitted by blood. The Kozup court held that the "remote possibility" of HIV transmission through blood transfusion could not, as a matter of law, have amounted to a "material risk." The court therefore ruled that the medical center owed no duty to disclose the risk and dismissed the plaintiff's informed consent claim.[35(p 1053)] In reaching its decision, the *Kozup* court emphasized that liability for nondisclosure is to be determined by "foresight, not hindsight." The focal point of the analysis must be the date when the plaintiff would have made the decision whether to accept the transfusion.[35(p 1054)]

Other courts have also ruled that there was insufficient information in the early 1980s to establish that there was material risk of HIV transmission from a blood transfusion. In *Gibson v. Methodist Hospital*, a Texas Court of Appeals found that no competent evidence was introduced to show that at the time of the March

1983 transfusion, there was a known material risk of contracting AIDS through blood transfusion.[13] A Wisconsin Court of Appeals also ruled that AIDS was not a material risk of blood transfusion in early 1983.[36]

However, in the middle 1980s other courts determined that the risk of HIV infection from blood transfusion was a material risk and should have been disclosed. The US District Court for the Western District of Texas ruled that the possibility in May 1984 of HIV transmission through transfusion could have influenced a reasonable person in making a decision to give or withhold consent.[37] When considering whether the risk of HIV transmission from blood transfusion was material in 1984, the US Court of Appeals for the Fifth Circuit attached great significance to the fact that AIDS is fatal.[38] An Ohio Court of Appeals ruled that the risk of transfusion-transmitted HIV was not too remote to be foreseeable in March 1985.[39]

Despite the fact that the risks of contracting HIV through transfusion have significantly diminished in recent years, public concern (including misperceptions and misinformation) remains high. Although health-care providers were often excused from liability in the early 1980s, a court examining materiality from the patient's perspective today would likely rule that health-care providers have a duty to disclose the risks of HIV (and other known transfusion-transmitted diseases) because of their severity, even though the chance of infection is remote.[1]

Proximate Cause

To prove an informed consent claim grounded in negligence, a plaintiff must establish not only that there was a duty to disclose transfusion risks, but also that the failure to disclose actually caused the injury (proximate cause). In other words, had the correct information been provided, the patient would have forgone the transfusion.

An informed consent claim must fail if a reasonable person would not have refused the transfusion. For example, in *Knight v. Department of the Army*, the plaintiff was in desperate need of cardiovascular surgery. The court dismissed the informed consent claim after finding it highly unlikely that the plaintiff would have withheld consent for the procedure on the basis of the transfusion risk.[37]

Special Transfusion-Related Issues of Informed Consent

Autologous Donation or Transfusion

The legal concepts discussed above apply even for patients scheduled for autologous donation and transfusion. Although there is little in the way of specific law, it is likely that a court would find that the risks associated with autologous transfusion are material and therefore would conclude that patients are entitled to disclosure of these risks. Autologous blood transfusion is generally considered safer than allogeneic transfusion, but certain risks are inherent in the donation, as well as in the storage and transfusion processes. These risks are different from those for allogeneic blood and should be explained to the patient. Directed donations—again with different risks—are also used as an alternative form of allogeneic blood transfusion. It is therefore prudent for a transfusion facility to develop appropriate informed consent procedures for patients electing autologous donations and directed donations.

Repetitive Transfusions

In situations in which therapy involves multiple transfusion procedures over an extended period, physicians may be faced with the issue of whether a single informed consent authorization from the patient is sufficient. For example, this issue could arise with patients undergoing a series of therapeutic apheresis procedures. While no court cases specifically addressing this issue were identified, general principles of informed consent law are applicable.

To be valid, consent for a medical procedure must be "informed." The patient must be given adequate information of the risks involved, or the consent is ineffective.[7] Thus if the risk to the patient of transfusion therapy varies over time, the new risk factors, logically, should be explained to the patient and additional consent obtained. This precept is especially applicable in situations in which the transfusions in question are administered as a part of separate therapies. However, since this area of law is unsettled, it is recommended that local counsel be consulted when an informed consent policy is developed for repetitive transfusion therapy.

Exceptions to Informed Consent Requirement

Emergency

Emergency situations provide exceptions to the requirement for advance consent. However, the law is complicated in cases in which emergencies arise after consent has occurred. If the emergency exception is invoked, the physician must be able to substantiate that the threat to the patient was immediate—not some future possibility—and even then, courts are reluctant to abrogate the patient's right to be informed and to choose appropriately.[40]

Waiver

Courts are reluctant to permit physicians to substitute their own judgment for that of the patient. If a physician decides to accept a waiver from the patient, documentation is key. The discussion should still include disclosure of all material risks, benefits, and alternatives that form the basis for the decision.[41]

Therapeutic Privilege

Some physicians choose to withhold information from patients pending definitive diagnostic or therapeutic interventions if they consider this course to be in the patients' best interest.[41] If the patient would have chosen to forgo the activity in light of the additional information obtained, the physician may be unable to justify to a jury why disclosure did not precede the interventional step. In situations in which the prognosis is poor, some patients may choose to forgo all medical treatments and opt to receive only palliation. It is the patient's right to choose, so therapeutic privilege should rarely be used. A better approach would be to work with an appropriate family member or mental health professional who can function as a surrogate decision-maker for the patient.

There are a few, relatively uncommon situations in which a physician may be excused from obtaining informed consent. For example, when risk is known to the patient or when the physician is unaware of a material risk and should not have been aware of it in the exercise of ordinary care, the physician will not be held liable for failing to obtain informed consent. Physicians rely on these exceptions at their own risk, however, since the issue of whether the risk was known to the patient and whether the physician should have been aware of the risk may be decided in distinct ways by different courts.

Conclusion

Considering the legal concepts articulated in this chapter, together with public perceptions of the transfusion risk and prevailing standards of practice, it is clear that informed consent should be obtained prior to administering transfusion therapy. This involves advising patients of all material risks of transfusion and obtaining their consent for all nonemergency procedures.

References

1. Lipton KS, Wolf EL. Medicolegal considerations. In: Petz LD, Swisher SN, Kleinman S, et al, eds. Clinical practice of transfu-

sion medicine, 3rd ed. New York: Churchill Livingstone, 1996:349-58.

2. Code of federal regulations. 21 CFR Section 50 et seq.
3. Food and Drug Administration. Waiver of informed consent requirements in certain emergency research. Fed Regist 1996;61:51531-3.
4. Cal. Health & Safety Code, Section 1645 (West 1995).
5. N.J. Stat. Ann. Section 26:2A-14 (West 1995).
6. 40 Pa. C.S.A. Sect. 1301.811.
7. Physician's duty to inform of risks, 88 ALR3d 1008.
8. *Traxler v. Vardy,* 16 Cal. Rptr.2d 297 (Cal. App. 1993).
9. *Hoffman v. Brandywine Hospital,* 661 A.2d 397 (Penn. Super. 1995).
10. *Jones v. Philadelphia College of Osteopathic Medicine,* 813 F. Suppl. (E.D. Pa. 1993).
11. Tex. Rev. Civ. Stat. Ann. Art. 4590i Section 6.02 (Vernon Supp. 1991).
12. Keeton WK, Dobbs DB, Keeton RE, Owen DG. Prosser and Keeton on the law of torts. 5th ed. St. Paul: West Publishing, 1984.
13. *Gibson v. Methodist Hospital,* 822 S.W.2d 95 (Tex. App. 1991).
14. *Smogor v. Enke,* 874 F.2d 295 (5th Cir. 1989).
15. Rosovsky FA. Consent to treatment, a practical guide. 2nd ed. Boston: Little, Brown and Co, 1990.
16. Greve PA Jr. Medical, ethical and legal issues associated with HIV. J Intravenous Nurs 1991;14(3 Suppl P):S30-5.
17. *Doe v. Lancaster General Hospital,* et al, No. 5033-1991 (Penn. Ct of Common Pleas Nov. 20, 1992).
18. *Goss v. Oklahoma Blood Institute,* 856 P2d 998 (Okl. App. 1990).
19. *Johnson v. Sears, Roebuck & Co,* 832 P.2d (N.M. App. 1992).
20. *Mafana v. Elie,* 439 N.E. 2d 1319 (Ill. App. 1982).
21. *Howell v. Spokane & Inland Empire Blood Bank,* 785 P.2d 815, 823 (Wash. 1990).
22. Comprehensive accreditation manual for hospitals. Oakbrook Terrace, IL: Joint Commission on Accreditation of Healthcare Organizations, 1995.

23. *Seley v. Searle & Co,* 67 Ohio St.2d 192, 423 N.E.2d 831 (1981).
24. *U.S. v. Charters,* 829 F.2d 479 (4th Cir. 1987).
25. *Palmer v. Biloxi Regional Medical Center, Inc,* 564 So.2d 1346 (Miss. 1990).
26. *Morgan v. Olds,* 417 N.W.2d 232 (Iowa App. 1988).
27. *J.V. v. State,* 516 So.2d 1133 (Fla. App. 1 Dist. 1987).
28. *In Re E.G.,* 5499 N.E. 2d 322 (Ill. 1989).
29. *Sawyer v. Methodist Hospital,* 522 F.2d (6th Cir. 1975).
30. *Salgo v. Leland Stanford Jr. University Board of Trustees,* 317 P.2d 170 (Cal. Dist. Ct. App. 1957).
31. *Canterbury v. Spence,* 464 F.2d (D.C. Cir. 1972).
32. *Arena v. Gingrich,* 305 Or. 1, 748 P.2d 547 (1988).
33. *McPherson v. Ellis,* 305 N.C. 730, 287 S.E.2d 892 (1982), overruled by N.C. Gen. Stat. Sect. 90-21.13.
34. *Cherry v. Herques,* 623 So.2d 131 (La. App. 1993).
35. *Kozup v. Georgetown University,* 663 F.Supp. 1048 (D.D.C. 1987), aff'd in part, 851 F.2d 437 (D.C. Cir. 1988).
36. *Ostrander v. Wisconsin Health Care Liability Insurance Plan,* et al, No. 89-0948-FY (Wisc. Ct. App. 1989).
37. *Knight v. Department of the Army,* 757 F.Supp. 790, 794 (W.D. Tex. 1991).
38. *Valdiviez v. U.S.,* 884 F.2d 196, 199-200 (5th Cir. 1989).
39. *Jeanne et al v. Hawkes Hospital of Mt. Carmel, et al,* No. 90AP-599 (Ohio Ct. App. 1991).
40. *Keogan v. Holy Family Hospital,* 95 Wash. 2d 306, 622 P.2d 1246 (1980).
41. Meisel A. The "exceptions" to the informed consent doctrine: Striking a balance between competing values in medical decision making. Wisconsin Law Review 1979:413.

Appendix 2-1. The Paul Gann Blood Safety Act[4]

1645. Standardized summary to surgical patient who may receive blood transfusion; Predonation

(a) Whenever there is a reasonable possibility, as determined by a physician and surgeon, that a blood transfusion may be necessary as a result of a medical or surgical procedure, the physician and surgeon, by means of a standardized written summary as most recently developed or revised by the State Department of Health Services pursuant to subdivision (e), shall inform the patient of the positive and negative aspects of receiving autologous blood and directed and nondirected homologous blood from volunteers. For purposes of this section, the term "autologous blood" includes, but is not limited to, predonation, intraoperative autologous transfusion, plasmapheresis, and hemodilution.

(b) The physician and surgeon shall note on the patient's medical record that the standardized written summary described in subdivision (e) was given to the patient.

(c) Subdivisions (a) and (b) shall not apply when medical contraindications or a life-threatening emergency exists.

(d) When there is no life-threatening emergency and there are no medical contraindications, the physician and surgeon shall allow adequate time prior to the procedure for predonation to occur. Notwithstanding this chapter, if a patient waives allowing adequate time prior to the procedure for predonation to occur, a physician and surgeon shall not incur any liability for his or her failure to allow adequate time prior to the procedure for predonation to occur.

(e) The State Department of Health Services shall develop and annually review, and if necessary revise, a standardized written summary which explains the advantages, disadvantages, risks, and descriptions of autologous blood, and directed and nondirected homologous blood from volunteer donors. These blood options shall include, but not be limited to, the blood options described in subdivision (a). The summary shall be written so as to be easily understood by a layperson.

(f) The Medical Board of California shall publish the standardized written summary prepared pursuant to subdivision (e) by the State Department of Health Services and shall distribute copies thereof, upon request, to physicians and surgeons. The Medical Board of California shall make the summary available for a fee not exceeding in the aggregate the actual costs to the State Department of Health Services and the Medical Board of California for developing, updating, publishing and distributing the summary. Physicians and surgeons shall purchase the written summary from the Medical Board of California for, or purchase or otherwise receive the written summary from any other entity for, distribution to their patients as specified in subdivision (a). Clinics, health facilities, and blood collection centers may purchase the summary if they desire.

(g) Any entity may reproduce the written summary prepared pursuant to subdivision (e) by the State Department of Health Services and distribute the written summary to physicians and surgeons.

HISTORY:
    Added State 1989 ch 1365 sec 2.
    Amended State 1990 ch 820 @ 1.
    Amended State 1991 ch 296 @ 1 (AB 787), effective August 1, 1991.

NOTES:
    AMENDMENTS:
    1990 Amendment: (1) Substituted "medical" for "surgical" after "result of a" is subd (a); (2) substituted "the procedure" for "surgery" after "time prior to" wherever it appears in subd (d); (3) amended subd (f) by (a) substituting "Medical Board of California" for "Board of Medical Quality Assurance" wherever it appears; (b) adding ", or purchase or otherwise receive the written summary

from any other entity for," after "of California for" in the third sentence; and (c) substituting the period for ", and" after "subdivision (a)"; and (4) added subd (g).

1991 Amendment: Amended the first sentence of subd (a) by (1) substituting "reasonable possibility, as determined by a physician and surgeon," for "possibility"; and (2) adding "or surgical".

COLLATERAL REFERENCES
B-W Cal Civ Prac, Torts @ 32:8.

Appendix 2-2. New Jersey Statute on Informed Consent[5]

26:2A-14. Surgery patient to be advised of options of receiving autologous, designated or homologous blood transfusion; exceptions; predonation of blood

a. Whenever a blood transfusion may be necessary during a surgical procedure, a physician or surgeon shall inform the surgery patient, prior to performing the surgical procedure, of the options of receiving autologous blood transfusions, designated blood transfusions or homologous blood transfusions.

b. The physician or surgeon who will perform the surgery shall note on the patient's medical record that the patient was advised of the opportunity to receive an autologous, designated or homologous blood transfusion, if a transfusion becomes necessary.

c. The physician or surgeon who will perform the surgery shall not be required to provide his patient with an explanation of the transfusion options pursuant to this section, if medical contraindications exist or the surgery is performed on an emergency basis.

d. If there are no medical contraindications or the surgery is not performed on an emergency basis, the physician or surgeon shall allow adequate time, prior to surgery, for predonation to occur. If the patient waives the option to predonate blood, the physician or surgeon shall not incur any liability for his failure to allow the predonation to occur.

Appendix 2-3. Pennsylvania Act on Informed Consent[6]

1301.811. Amending the act of October 15, 1975 (P.L. 390, No. 111), entitled "an act relating to medical and health related malpractice insurance, prescribing the powers and duties of the insurance department; providing for a joint underwriting plan; the arbitration panels for health care, compulsory screening of claims; collateral sources requirement; limitation on contingent fee compensation; establishing a catastrophe loss fund; and prescribing penalties," further providing for definitions, for statute of limitations, for professional liability insurance and the medical professional liability catastrophe loss fund, for person, corporation, university or other educational institution, facility, institution or other entity licensed or approved by the commonwealth to provide health care or professional medical services as a physician, (an osteopathic physician or surgeon,) a certified nurse midwife, a podiatrist, hospital, nursing home, birth center, and except as to section 701(A), an officer, employee or agent of any of them acting in the course and scope of (his) employment.

"Immediate family" means a parent, spouse or child or an adult sibling residing in the same household.

"Informed consent" means for the purposes of this act and of any proceedings arising under the provisions of this act, the consent of a patient to the performance of (health care services by a physician or podiatrist; provided, that prior to the consent having been given, the physician or podiatrist has informed the patient of the nature of the proposed procedure or treatment and of those risks and alternatives to treatment or diagnosis that a reasonable patient would consider material to the decision whether or not to undergo treatment or diagnosis. No physician or podiatrist shall be liable for a failure to obtain an informed consent in the event of an emergency which prevents consulting the patient. No physician or podiatrist shall be liable for failure to obtain an informed consent if it is established by a preponderance of the evidence that furnishing the information in question to the patient would have resulted in a seriously adverse effect on the patient or on the therapeutic process to the material detriment of the patient's health.) A procedure in accordance with section 811-A.

Section 811-A. Informed consent.

(A) Except in emergencies, a physician owes a duty to a patient to obtain the informed consent of the patient or the patient's authorized representative prior to conducting the following procedures:

(1) Performing surgery, including the related administration of anesthesia.

(2) Administering radiation or chemotherapy.

(3) Administering a blood transfusion.

(4) Inserting a surgical device or appliance.

(5) Administering an experimental medication, using an experimental device or using an approved medication or device in an experimental manner.

(B) Consent is informed if the patient has been given a description of a procedure set forth in subsection (A) and the risks and alternatives that a reasonably prudent patient would require to make an informed decision as to that procedure. The physician shall be entitled to present evidence of the description of that procedure and those risks and alternatives that a physician acting in accordance with accepted medical standards of medical practice would provide.

(C) Expert testimony is required to determine whether the procedure constituted the type of procedure set forth in subsection (A) and to identify the risks of that procedure, the alternatives to that procedure and the risks of these alternatives.

(D) A physician is liable for failure to obtain the informed consent only if the patient proves that receiving such information would have been a substantial factor in the patient's decision whether to undergo a procedure set forth in subsection (A).

In: Stowell, CP, ed.
Informed Consent for Blood Transfusion
Bethesda, MD: American Association of Blood Banks, 1997

3

Infectious Risks of Transfusion

Steven Kleinman, MD

The major risks of blood transfusion are due to the transmission of infectious agents, particularly viruses. Since the risks of transfusion-transmitted infection are currently very low and continue to decrease as technology advances, it is difficult to accurately measure and quantitate these risks.[1-2] Consequently, risk estimates have been obtained with mathematical modeling techniques applied to data sets from infectious disease testing of blood donors or follow-up investigations of selected transfusion recipients.[3-7]

Transfusion-Transmitted Diseases

The current risks of transfusion-transmitted infection, expressed per unit of blood received, are given in Table 3-1. These risks are expressed per unit of transfused blood rather than per patient; this allows the more precise computation of risk for a given patient (ie, by multiplying the per-unit risk times the number of units transfused). For the most important transfusion-transmissible agents—human immunodeficiency virus (HIV) and hepatitis C virus (HCV)—the per-unit risk is the same for each type of blood component transfused (red cells, platelets, fresh frozen plasma, cryoprecipitate). In contrast, for human T-cell lymphotropic virus types I

Steven Kleinman, MD, Transfusion Medicine Consultant, Victoria, British Columbia, Canada

Table 3-1. Per-Unit Risk of Transmitting Infectious Agents Through Blood Transfusion (as of December 1995)

Infectious Agents	Per-Unit Risk Estimate	Reference
Human immunodeficiency virus	1 in 545,000-733,000	(Refs 5,8,9)
Human T-cell lymphotropic virus, I and II*	1 in 50,000-100,000	(Refs 1,2,10)
Hepatitis B virus	1 in 66,000-200,000	(Refs 1,2,8,10)
Hepatitis C virus	1 in 5000[†]	(Ref 6)
Other (bacteria, parasites)	< 1 in 1 million	(Ref 11)

*Only platelets and red cells stored less than 14 days will transmit infection to recipients.[12,13]

[†]Estimate based upon existence of chronic carrier state undetected by current assays; estimate of risk due solely to window period transmission is approximately 1 in 103,000.[7,8]

and II (HTLV-I/II), there is no risk of transmission from acellular blood components (fresh frozen plasma or cryoprecipitate), since HTLV is highly leukocyte-associated.[12]

Despite the fact that each donated unit of blood is tested for markers of viral infection, there are at least three potential reasons why transmission of viral agents still occurs. The leading factor is the inability to obtain a positive test result during the early stages of infection, known as the "window period." For example, an individual exposed to HIV does not develop the HIV antibody identified in the HIV test until some defined period has elapsed (this is estimated to average approximately 22 days with current HIV antibody tests).[14] However, if such an individual were to donate blood during this window period, his or her transfused unit would be capable of transmitting HIV infection. The HIV-1 antigen test has reduced, but not eliminated, the window period.

A second factor contributing to transfusion-transmitted infection is the existence of the chronic carrier who persistently tests negative on the donor screening tests. For example, there is evidence that some HCV-infected individuals may carry the virus, but it is undetectable by the current antibody tests.[15] Similarly, HTLV-II in some chronic carriers is not detected by current HTLV-I antibody tests.[16] A third factor that could theoretically contribute to transfusion-transmitted infection is laboratory error in performing screening tests; this is thought to be extremely rare.

Human Immunodeficiency Virus

In 1989 American Red Cross investigators published a study estimating that the risk of HIV infection from blood transfusion was 1 in 153,000 units.[4] Since HIV antibody screening tests have markedly improved in the 1990s, it is not surprising that more recent risk estimates are considerably lower. A risk estimate of 1 in 225,000 per unit, derived from an unpublished study by the Centers for Disease Control and Prevention (CDC), was cited in a 1992 *New England Journal of Medicine* editorial.[10] More recently, CDC investigators have estimated the risk of HIV infection to be 1 in 450,000-660,000 units[5]; a similar analysis performed by a group of investigators from the Retrovirus Epidemiology Donor Study (REDS) yielded an estimate of 1 in 493,000.[8] With the implementation of HIV-1 p24 antigen testing, it has been predicted that the estimated risk of HIV infection from transfusion will be decreased by 25%, yielding a new risk estimate of 1 in 545,000-733,000 units.

Hepatitis C Virus

In the early 1990s, published risk estimates for HCV transmission by blood transfusion were 1 in 3300 units; this estimate was derived at a time when HCV antibody testing was performed with a first-generation, C100, antibody assay.[10,17] Since 1992 blood banks have performed HCV antibody testing with a more sensitive multiantigen assay. It has been estimated that the risk of transfusion-transmitted HCV infection may have fallen to approximately 1 in 5000 per unit with the introduction of this improved testing.[1,6] These estimates are all based upon the premise that transmission can occur from chronic HCV carriers who are not identified by current antibody tests; this phenomenon was reported by CDC investigators who found that such carriers may represent 10% of HCV-infected people.[15] There has been no further confirmation of this initial report, however, making it difficult to establish the extent of this phenomenon. HCV transmission from recent acute infection in the window period has been estimated to occur at a rate of 1 in 103,000 per unit.[7,8]

Human T-Cell Lymphotropic Virus

The risk of HTLV-I infection by blood transfusion is thought to be very low. However, a closely related retrovirus, HTLV-II, may be more commonly transmitted by blood transfusion. Current screening tests for HTLV infection are designed to detect antibody formed to HTLV-I and will detect some but not all individuals infected with HTLV-II because of cross-reactivity of antibodies to the two viruses. The combined risk of HTLV-I/II infection has been estimated as 1 in 50,000-100,000 per unit.[1,2]

Hepatitis B Virus

The risk of hepatitis B infection from blood transfusion is extremely low because of the simultaneous use of two hepatitis B assays—hepatitis B surface antigen (HBsAg) and hepatitis B core antibody (anti-HBc). By use of these two tests, hepatitis B transmission is prevented unless the donor is in the early incubation (window) phase of hepatitis B infection. This risk has not been well-characterized by prospective serologic monitoring of transfusion recipients. On the basis of reports of clinically apparent posttransfusion hepatitis B infection, the risk has been estimated as 1 in 200,000.[1,2] More recently, REDS investigators have used data from HBsAg seroconverting blood donors to derive a per-unit risk estimate for hepatitis B transmission of 1 in 66,000.

Bacterial Infection

Recently, there has been renewed concern about the risk of transmitting bacterial infection by blood transfusion.[18] It is known that septic transfusion reactions are more frequent with transfused platelet concentrates than with red cells; platelets are stored for up to 5 days at room temperature and provide a better growth medium for bacteria than do refrigerated red cells. Data indicate that fatal transfusion reactions due to bacterial sepsis occur at a rate of less than 1 in a million.[11] It is more difficult to assess the rate of significant morbidity from bacterially infected units. Although laboratory data indicate that bacteria can be cultured from up to 0.3% of platelet concentrates, the significance of these findings is unclear. It is unknown whether these in-vitro data represent true contamination of the unit; furthermore, it is not known whether small amounts of transfused bacteria cause recipient morbidity.[11,19]

Progression of Transfusion-Transmitted Infection to Disease

Recipients who acquire HIV infection from blood transfusion progress to AIDS at a rate similar to that of others infected with HIV. Therefore, persons infected with HIV from blood transfusion will eventually develop AIDS if they survive the underlying disease that necessitated their transfusion.[20] Disease associations arising from HTLV-I or HTLV-II infection are much less frequent than from HIV. It has been estimated that 4% of individuals infected with HTLV-I at birth progress to adult T-cell leukemia, usually after an incubation period of at least 20-30 years.[21] A neurologic syndrome, HTLV-I-associated myelopathy has been estimated to occur in 0.25% of persons infected with this virus af-

ter an incubation period of months to years.[22] A similar neurologic syndrome caused by HTLV-II has also been documented;
however, there is no evidence linking HTLV-II infection with
adult T-cell leukemia.[23]

The natural history of transfusion-acquired HCV is similar to
that of HCV acquired through other modes of transmission. Approximately 50% of patients develop chronic elevations of liver
enzymes, and 10% of these will develop microscopic evidence of
cirrhosis.[24,25] The symptoms of a small percentage of chronically
infected patients are severe enough to require treatment. Anecdo-
tal reports of significant morbidity and of mortality have been described, and persistent evidence of chronic biochemical
abnormalities have been documented in approximately 30% of
patients on 20-year follow-up.[26] However, this same study failed
to document any excess mortality on 18-year follow-up in a large
group of patients with posttransfusion HCV infection.[27]

References

1. Kleinman S, Busch MP. General overview of transfusion transmitted infections. In: Petz LD, Swisher SN, Kleinman S, et al,
   eds. In: Clinical practice of transfusion medicine. New York:
   Churchill Livinqston, 1995:809-21.
2. Dodd RY. Adverse consequences of blood transfusion: Quantitative risk estimates. In: Nance ST, ed. Blood supply: Risk,
   perceptions and prospects for the future. Bethesda, MD:
   American Association of Blood Banks, 1993:1-24.
3. Busch MP, Eble BE, Khayam-Bashi H, et al. Evaluation of
   screened blood donations for human immunodeficiency virus
   type 1 infection by culture and DNA amplification of pooled
   cells. N Engl J Med 1991;325:1-5.
4. Cumming PD, Wallace EL, Schorr JB, Dodd RY. Exposure of
   patients to human immunodeficiency virus through the transfusion of blood components that test antibody-negative. N
   Engl J Med 1989;321:941-6.

5. Lackritz EM, Satten GA, Aberle-Grasse J, et al. Estimated risk of HIV transmission by screened blood in the United States. N Engl J Med 1995;333:1721-5.
6. Kleinman S, Busch M, Holland P. Post-transfusion hepatitis C virus infection (letter). N Engl J Med 1992:327(22):1601-2.
7. Schreiber GB, Busch MP, Gilcher RO, et al. Incidence rates of infectious disease markers in repeat blood donors (abstract). Transfusion 1994;34(Suppl):71S.
8. Schreiber GB, Busch, MP, Kleinman SH, Korelitz JJ. The risk of transfusion transmitted viral infections. N Engl J Med 1996;334(26):1685-90.
9. Centers for Disease Control and Prevention. US Public Health Service guidelines for testing and counseling blood and plasma donors for human immunodificiency virus, type 1 antigen. MMWR 1996;45(RR-2):1-9.
10. Dodd RY. The risk of transfusion-transmitted infection (editorial). N Engl J Med 1992;327:419-21.
11. Wagner SJ, Friedman LI, Dodd RY. Transfusion-associated bacterial sepsis. Clin Microbiol Rev 1994;7:290-302.
12. Okochi K, Satao H, Hinuma Y. A retrospective study on transmission of adult T-cell leukemia virus by blood transfusion: Seroconversion in recipients. Vox Sang 1984;46:245-53.
13. Donegan E, Lee H, Operskalski EA, et al. Transfusion transmission of retroviruses: Human T-lymphotropic viruses types I and II compared with human immunodeficiency virus type I. Transfusion 1994;34:478-83.
14. Busch MP, Lee LLL, Satten GA, et al. Time course of detection of viral and serologic markers preceding human immunodeficiency virus type 1 seroconversion: Implications for screening of blood and tissue donors. Transfusion 1995;35:91-7.
15. Alter MJ, Margolis HS, Krawczynski K, et al. The natural history of community-acquired hepatitis C in the United States. N Engl J Med 1992;327:1899-905.
16. Hjelle B, Wilson C, Cyrus S, et al. Human T-cell leukemia virus type II infection frequently goes undetected in contemporary U.S. blood donors. Blood 1993;81:1641-4.

17. Donohue JG, Munoz A, Ness PM, et al. The declining risk of post-transfusion hepatitis C virus infection. N Engl J Med 1992;327:369-73.
18. Blajchman MA. Transfusion-associated bacterial sepsis: The phoenix rises yet again (editorial). Transfusion 1994;34:940.
19. Goldman M. Blajchman MA. Blood product-associated bacterial sepsis. Transfus Med Rev 1991;5:73-83.
20. Brookmeyer R. Reconstruction and future trends of the AIDS epidemic in the United States. Science 1991;253:37-42.
21. Murphy EL, Hanchard B, Figueroa JP, et al. Modeling the risk of adult T-cell leukemia/lymphoma in persons infected with human T-lymphotropic virus type I. Int J Cancer 1989;43: 250-3.
22. Kaplan JE, Osame M, Kubota H, et al. The risk of development of HTLV-I-associated myelopathy/tropical spastic paraparesis among persons infected with HTLV-I. J Acquir Immune Defic Syndr Hum Retrovirol 1990;3:1096-101.
23. Murphy EL, Fridey J, Smith JW, et al. HTLV-associated myelopathy in a cohort of HTLV-I and HTLV-II infected blood donors. Neurology 1997 (in press).
24. Alter HJ. To C or not to C: These are the questions. Blood 1995;85:1681-95.
25. Alter HJ. You'll wonder where the yellow went: A 15-year retrospective of posttransfusion hepatitis. In: Moore SB, ed. Transfusion-transmitted viral diseases. Arlington, VA: American Association of Blood Banks, 1987:53.
26. Seeff LB. Natural history of viral hepatitis, type C. Semin Gastrointest Dis 1995;6:20-7.
27. Seeff LB, Buskell-Bales Z, Wright EC, et al. Long-term mortality after transfusion-associated non-A, non-B hepatitis. N Engl J Med 1992;327:1906-11 [comment 1992;327:1949-50].

In: Stowell, CP, ed.
Informed Consent for Blood Transfusion
Bethesda, MD: American Association of Blood Banks, 1997

4

Noninfectious Complications of Transfusion with Allogeneic Blood Components

Linda A. Chambers, MD

Patients and their families may be very concerned about transfusion-transmitted human immunodeficiency virus (HIV). However, a complete and responsible presentation of transfusion risks includes infectious risks other than HIV, as well as consequences of transfusion that do not involve transmission of any infectious agents. Perhaps even more than for infectious risks, the consequences and relative importance of noninfectious complications are highly patient-specific. Therefore, this discussion of the noninfectious risks of allogeneic transfusion also identifies the types of patients and circumstances in which the risk is of unusual consequence or magnitude.

Some risks are well-established, while others are controversial and under investigation. Therefore, this presentation may not be complete. It can, however, be used to remind those making treatment decisions of the noninfectious transfusion complications that might be of particular relevance for a specific patient.

Linda A. Chambers, MD, Chief of Clinical Pathology and Medical Director, Transfusion Service, Children's Hospital, Columbus, Ohio

Transfusion Reactions

Reactions during or soon after transfusion, by any of the common mechanisms (allergic, hemolytic, septic, or white-cell-related), are usually mild and easily treated. In each category, however, are examples of more serious, even life-threatening, presentations. Hypersensitivity reactions to donor plasma immunoglobulin (Ig) A in IgA-deficient patients with anti-IgA can be frankly anaphylactic. While the typical white-cell-related reaction consists of fever and chills, transfusion-related acute lung injury precipitates respiratory failure, often requiring temporary ventilator support.

The most likely type of transfusion reaction varies predictably with the component transfused.[1] Allergic reactions to plasma proteins are more likely to occur with fresh frozen plasma (FFP) transfusion. White-cell-related reactions are expected during granulocyte transfusion. Septic reactions are a particular risk with components that have been manipulated in an open system (recovered blood, pooled components) and with platelets, as the room temperature storage offers more types of trace bacterial contaminants the opportunity to proliferate.[2]

Patient and clinical characteristics also influence the transfusion reaction rate. Because preexisting antibodies directed at IgE, red-cell, and white-cell antigens are more prevalent, the atopic, multitransfused or multiparous patient may be at increased risk for all varieties of nonseptic reactions.[3,4] Patients with longstanding exposure to latex from medical devices or as health-care workers, can develop severe latex allergies so that, at least theoretically, transfusion through latex-connected tubing could precipitate anaphylaxis. The risk of a hemolytic transfusion reaction is undoubtedly increased when a transfusion is performed in relatively uncontrolled settings, such as when a patient receives an emergency transfusion of uncrossmatched red cells or when a patient is transfused following complicated compatibility testing, eg, for warm autoimmune hemolytic anemia.[4,5]

Antibody Formation

Each of the cellular constituents of blood components (red cells, white cells, and platelets) carries its own foreign-donor antigens, which can be immunogenic. While antibody formation per se is usually a nonpathologic response, the presence of antibodies can complicate current and future medical therapy, increase the risk of transfusion reactions, and adversely affect subsequent pregnancies.

The frequency of red cell antibody formation differs among patient groups and may correlate only loosely with the total number of red cells transfused.[6] Women with autoimmune diseases tend to make red cell antibodies readily.[7] Infants and children, even when transfused repeatedly for conditions such as sickle cell anemia, infrequently become sensitized.[8] Patients with malignancies who receive chemotherapy are sufficiently immune-suppressed that red cell antibody formation is uncommon. Indeed, the rate of anti-D formation in Rh-negative oncology patients transfused repeatedly with Rh-positive platelets and granulocyte concentrates has been reported to be less than 20%.[9]

If a patient who is dependent on red cell transfusions (eg, for Fanconi's anemia, sickle cell disease, α-thalassemia) becomes sensitized to multiple red cell antibodies, locating appropriate antigen-negative units and confirming compatibility become increasingly difficult. Occasionally, some desirable therapies (bone marrow transplantation, exchange transfusion) are simply not feasible. Emergency transfusion of uncrossmatched blood becomes a very high-risk option, and the likelihood of acute or delayed hemolytic transfusion reactions is substantial.

In contrast to red cell antibody formation, sensitization to platelet-specific (non-HLA) antigens can be pathologic when the antibody (usually anti-HPA-1) displays a broad reactivity with both the transfused HPA-1-positive platelets and the patient's endogenous HP-A1-negative platelets. The resulting condition—posttransfusion purpura—has a high mortality with few effective treatment options; fortunately, it is rare.[10]

More problematic from a clinical perspective is the effect of platelet antigen sensitization on responsiveness to subsequent platelet transfusions. Both platelet-specific and HLA-antigen-directed antibodies from prior transfusion or pregnancy cause early clearance of transfused platelets, recognizable clinically as platelet refractoriness.[11-13] There are numerous immunologic and nonimmunologic causes of refractoriness—including conditions common in platelet transfusion recipients—such as fever, infection, and amphotericin treatment.[14] As with red cell component selection for transfusion-dependent, red-cell-sensitized patients, providing therapeutically-effective platelet transfusions for patients with platelet-reactive antibodies may be complicated, expensive, or nearly impossible. Aggressive therapies such as bone marrow transplantation may have a much higher predicted mortality when availability of effective platelet transfusion is limited.

HLA sensitization from transfusion may similarly make it more difficult to locate appropriate kidneys for renal transplantation and donors for allogeneic bone marrow transplantation because HLA antibodies limit the choice of compatible organs. Pre-existing HLA sensitization may set the stage for rejection of nonrenal solid organ transplants and for delayed or failed engraftment of transplanted bone marrow.[15]

In females of childbearing potential, platelet, red-cell, or white-cell antibodies can cross the placenta and cause cytopenias in the fetus and newborn; platelet antibodies can cause neonatal isoimmune thrombocytopenia, red-cell antibodies can cause hemolytic disease of the newborn and white-cell antibodies can cause neonatal neutropenia.[16-18]

Physical Effects

Rapid or large-volume transfusion can lead to fluid overload, particularly in patients with a small intravascular volume relative to the "standard" transfusion dose, limited left ventricular function or compromised renal function. The elderly and those with an unstable cardiovascular status may have especially poor tolerance for the intravascular volume expansion and fluid shifts associated with transfusion.[19]

Blood components are significantly cooler than body core temperature, particularly red cells issued from refrigerator storage and transfused promptly. Even with use of a blood warmer, depending on the starting temperature of the component and the flow rate through the heat exchange system, red cell components are below 30 C, or even 20 C, as they enter the patient's circulation.[20] Rapid infusion of large amounts of blood relative to the size of the patient can lower the core temperature enough to increase metabolic demand or even induce cardiac arrhythmias. In the critically unstable patient or a patient, such as a small infant, who is physiologically unable to compensate, transfusion-induced hypothermia may be harmful.[21] Hypothermia—even local cooling at the site of transfusion—should also be avoided in patients with significant cold agglutinins or cryoglobulins because of the risk of complement activation and vasculitis.[22]

Another type of physical effect of transfusion that can be clinically troublesome is simple dilution of peripheral blood constituents lacking in the transfused component. Appreciable dilution obviously requires a high total transfusion volume. As a rough guide, transfusion of one total blood volume with use of a component deficient in a given constituent reduces the level in the patient to about 70% of the starting value. Two blood volumes leaves about half (70% of 70%) of the patient's peripheral blood constituents. This means the count or level will be about half of the starting value. Certainly, coincident processes affect the actual washout kinetics. Release of platelets from the spleen abates the reduction in platelet count, while disseminated intravascular coagulation leading to consumption of coagulation proteins may magnify the washout effect.

In general however, dilutional thrombocytopenia and dilutional coagulation protein deficiency should be suspected if abnormal hemostasis develops in a patient receiving transfusion in excess of two total blood volumes.[23] High-risk clinical settings include not only during massive transfusion in trauma resuscitation, but also during cardiopulmonary bypass and extracorporeal membrane oxygenation, following large-volume recovery and reinfusion of washed red cells, and during neonatal whole blood exchange.[24]

Chemical Effects

When infused in large amounts over short periods, the citrate anticoagulant in blood components, which prevents coagulation protein activation by binding the needed calcium cofactor, can lower the transfusion recipient's plasma levels of ionized calcium below the normal physiologic range. The consequent tingling, twitching, and cardiac arrhythmias may be only bothersome symptoms or clinically problematic, especially in complex medical settings such as trauma resuscitation and surgery, where hypocalcemia is only one of many possible factors compromising cardiac function.[25] Routine calcium supplementation during transfusion is not required. However, with the onset of findings typical of hypocalcemia, slowing the transfusion rate to permit the hepatic metabolism of citrate to catch up may be required. Blood components containing relatively large amounts of citrate, such as FFP, are more likely to cause this complication. Plasma exchange—plasmapheresis with FFP replacement—combines large-volume transfusion with a high-risk component, so citrate reactions and hypocalcemia symptoms are quite common.[26] Patients with poor or no hepatic function, such as those undergoing hepatic transplantation, may be particularly vulnerable, since they are unable to rapidly metabolize the citrate.

Hyperkalemia or potassium toxicity with cardiac arrhythmias is an uncommon complication of red cell transfusion. During storage, red cells lose intracellular potassium in exchange for sodium, so the noncellular supernatant levels of potassium increase progressively. This process is accelerated in red cells that have been gamma-irradiated to prevent transfusion-associated graft-vs-host disease (GVHD).[27] While the concentration in the supernatant fluid may reach very high levels (25 mEq/L or more) in older units, the actual number of milliequivalents of potassium delivered with a typical transfusion dose is unremarkable. Once distributed throughout the total body water and exchanged for other electrolytes at the red cell membrane, the potassium administered with routine transfusion volumes of red cells does not change serum levels in the patient.

When the potassium level is very high *and* the transfusion volume is very high, frank hyperkalemia and potassium toxicity can develop, sometimes with a fatal outcome. Therefore, patients at special risk for potassium toxicity from red cell transfusion include 1) patients who receive rapid, large-volume transfusions (defined in proportion to patient total blood volume) especially during cardiac surgery, 2) patients with preexisting potassium metabolism problems (renal failure, acidosis), and 3) patients who are given components that have been gamma-irradiated and stored.[27,28]

Because each unit of packed red cells contains approximately 250 mg of iron in hemoglobin and because nonbleeding patients conserve and recycle iron from senescent red cells, chronic red cell transfusion invariably leads to iron overload, with deposition in organs such as the liver.[29] Over time, the accumulated iron results in tissue damage, scarring, and dysfunction (hemochromatosis). Chelation with drugs that extract and solubilize excess iron to permit excretion is an effective but lengthy treatment.

Immunologic Effects

Transfusion can cause GVHD when the immunologically competent donor lymphocytes in the blood component engraft, proliferate, and attack recipient tissues.[30,31] The risk may be increased with components containing the largest numbers of lymphocytes, such as granulocyte concentrates and fresh whole blood. In order for donor lymphocytes to successfully engraft, the recipient must be either immune-incompetent or immunologically "blind" to the foreign lymphocytes because of HLA similarity between the donor and patient. Transfusion-associated GVHD is a topic of considerable interest, and the details of identifying patient groups at risk, for whom gamma-irradiation of cellular components is indicated, is beyond the scope of this discussion. However at a minimum, patients with known or suspected cellular lymphocytic immunodeficiency and patients receiving transfusions that are closely tissue-matched or from a biologic relative should be considered at risk for this rare but invariably fatal complication of transfusion.

There is convincing laboratory evidence that transfusion leads to profound immediate changes and more subtle long-term changes in aspects of the immune system. Also under active investigation is whether these effects cause or complicate disease. Allogeneic transfusion may increase the risk of postoperative infections, progression of HIV-related diseases, and recurrence of some malignancies, presumably as a result of the immune system effects.[32,33] The magnitude and relative importance of the effect, if any, remain to be elucidated.

Summary

A complete presentation of transfusion risks during a discussion to elicit informed consent includes the noninfectious risks that may be particularly relevant to the clinical circumstance. These risks may be minimal or play a major role in a proper risk/benefit assessment, depending on the patient's illness, treatment plans, and prognosis as well as the transfusion component, expected volume, and rate. Table 4-1 lists the noninfectious risks of transfusion, and a quick review with a particular patient in mind will help to ensure that none are overlooked.

References

1. Heddle NM, Klama LN, Griffith L, et al. A prospective study to identify the risk factors associated with acute reactions to platelet and red cell transfusions. Transfusion 1993;33:794-7.
2. Morrow JF, Braine HG, Kickler TS, et al. Septic reactions to platelet transfusions. A persistent problem. JAMA 1991;266:555-8.

Table 4-1. Noninfectious Transfusion Risks and Adverse Consequences

1. Transfusion reactions
   a. Usually mild
      Allergic reactions to blood proteins
      Febrile nonhemolytic
      Delayed hemolytic
      Allergic reactions to storage or transfusion equipment*
   b. Potentially severe
      Hemolytic
      Severe allergic and anaphylactic
      Transfusion-acquired acute lung injury
      Septic shock*

2. Alloantibody formation
   a. To red cell antigens
   b. To platelet-specific antigens
      Posttransfusion purpura
      Neonatal isoimmune thrombocytopenia
   c. To HLA antigens
      Platelet refractoriness

3. Physical effects*
   a. Fluid overload
   b. Hypothermia
   c. Dilutional coagulopathy

4. Chemical effects*
   a. Hypocalcemia
   b. Hyperkalemia
   c. Iron overload, hemochromatosis

5. Immunologic effects
   a. Graft-vs-host disease
   b. Immune suppression and dysregulation

*These risks occur with both allogeneic and autologous transfusion. The other noninfectious risks are restricted to allogeneic transfusions, whether from the general blood supply or directed donations.

3. Fluit CRMG, Kunst VAJM, Krenthe-Schonk AM. Incidence of red cell antibodies after multiple blood transfusion. Transfusion 1990;30:532-5.
4. Ness PM, Shirey RS, Thomas SK, et al. The differentiation of delayed serologic and delayed hemolysis transfusion reactions: Incidence, long-term serologic findings, and clinical significance. Transfusion 1990;30:688-93.
5. Harrison CR, Hayes TC, Trow LL, et al. Intravascular hemolytic transfusion reaction without detectable antibodies: A case report and review of literature. Vox Sang 1986;51:96-101.
6. Lasky LC, Rose RR, Polesky HF. Incidence of antibody formation and positive direct antiglobulin tests in a multitransfused hemodialysis population. Transfusion 1984;24:198-200.
7. Ramsey G, Smietana SJ. Multiple or uncommon red cell alloantibodies in women: Associated with autoimmune disease. Transfusion 1995;35:582-6.
8. Rosse WF, Gallagher D, Kinney TR, et al. Transfusion and alloimmunization in sickle cell disease. Blood 1990;76:1431-7.
9. Baldwin ML, Ness PM, Scott D, et al. Alloimmunization to D antigen and HLA in D-negative immunosuppressed oncology patients. Transfusion 1988;28:330-3.
10. Chaplin H, Aster RH, Morgan LK, et al. First example of familial posttransfusion purpura in two Pl^{A1}-negative sisters. Transfusion 1988;28:326-9.
11. Kickler T, Kennedy SD, Braine HG. Alloimmunization to platelet-specific antigens on glycoproteins IIb-IIIa and Ib/IX in multiply-transfused thrombocytopenic patients. Transfusion 1990;30:622-5.
12. Kickler TS. The challenge of platelet alloimmunization: Management and prevention. Transfus Med Rev 1990;4(Suppl 1):8-18.
13. Hoard JE, Perkins HA. The natural history of alloimmunization to platelets. Transfusion 1978;18:496-503.
14 Bishop JF, McGrath K, Wolf MM, et al. Clinical factors influencing the efficacy of pooled platelet transfusions. Blood 1988;71:383-7.

15. Stroncek DF. Results of bone marrow transplants from unrelated donors. Transfusion 1992;32:180-9.
16. Cartron J, Tchernia G, Celton JL, et al. Alloimmune neonatal neutropenia. Am J Pediatr Hematol Oncol 1991;13:21-5.
17. Kiefel V, Schechter Y, Atias D, et al. Neonatal alloimmune thrombocytopenia due to anti-Br[b] (HPA-5a). Vox Sang 1991; 60:244-5.
18. Bowman JM. Treatment options for the fetus with alloimmune hemolytic disease. Transfus Med Rev 1990;4:191-207.
19. Harrison CR, Sawyer PR. Special issues in transfusion medicine. Clin Lab Med 1992;12:743-57.
20. Uhl L, Pacini D, Kruskall MS. A comparative study of blood warmer performance. Anesthesiology 1992;77:1022-8.
21. Nolan TE, Gallup DG. Massive transfusion: A current review. Obstet Gynecol Surv 1991;46:289-95.
22. Iverson KV, Huestis DW. Blood warming: Current applications and techniques. Transfusion 1991;31:558-71.
23. Counts RB, Haisch C, Simon TL, et al. Hemostasis in massively transfused trauma patients. Ann Surg 1979;190:91-9.
24. Kern FH, Morano NJ, Sears JJ, et al. Coagulation defects in neonates during cardiopulmonary bypass. Ann Thorac Surg 1992;54:541-6.
25. Wilson RF, Binkley LE, Sabo FM, et al. Electrolyte and acid-base changes with massive blood transfusions. Am Surg 1992;58:535-44.
26. Robinson A. Hazards of apheresis and the U.K. approach to guidelines. Transfus Sci 1990;11:305-8.
27. Brugnara C, Churchill WH. Effect of irradiation on red cell cation content and transport. Transfusion 1992;32:246-52.
28. Hall TL, Barnes A, Miller JR, et al. Neonatal mortality following transfusion of red blood cells with high potassium. Transfusion 1993;33:606-9.
29. Conrad ME. Sickle cell disease and hemochromatosis. Am J Hematol 1991;38:150-2.
30. Anderson KC, Weinstein HJ. Transfusion-associated graft-versus-host disease. N Engl J Med 1990;323:315-320.

31. Davey RJ. Transfusion-associated graft-versus-host disease and the irradiation of blood components. Immunol Invest 1995;24:431-4.
32. Blumberg N, Triulzi DJ, Heal JM. Transfusion-induced immunomodulation and its clinical consequences. Transfus Med Rev 1990;4:24-35.
33. Brunson ME, Alexander JW. Mechanisms of transfusion-induced immunosuppression. Transfusion 1990;30:651-8.

In: Stowell, CP, ed.
Informed Consent for Blood Transfusion
Bethesda, MD: American Association of Blood Banks, 1997

5

The Benefits of Transfusion

Christopher P. Stowell, MD, PhD

An important component of the informed consent process is the explanation to the patient of the potential benefit that might be expected from a procedure or a therapeutic agent. The expected benefits of medications and procedures have frequently been the subject of clinical trials and can often be explained on the basis of documented clinical experience in quantitative terms. The discussion of the benefits of transfusion is not generally so straightforward. Very little information comparable to that obtained from clinical trials is usually available to the physician attempting to explain the benefits anticipated from transfusion. Our understanding of the efficacy of transfusion relies rather heavily on a general knowledge of physiology, practice traditions, and personal experience with patients. Although there is literature that addresses the indications for transfusion, the focus tends to be on 1) the decision-making process or 2) the analysis of various transfusion strategies—such as the use of transfusion "triggers" or a comparison of therapeutic and prophylactic transfusion algorithms. The benefits of transfusion are often only obliquely demonstrated in these studies.

In many transfusion situations that lack of extensive published documentation of efficacy, the discussion of benefits with an indi-

Christopher P. Stowell, MD, PhD, Director, Blood Transfusion Service, Massachusetts General Hospital, and Department of Pathology, Harvard Medical School, Boston, Massachusetts

vidual patient must focus on the specific, desired clinical outcome the transfusion is intended to achieve. This chapter discusses some of the considerations that must be addressed during the discussion between physician and patient.

Preparing to Discuss the Benefits of Transfusion with the Patient

Even before initiating a discussion of the benefits of transfusion with the patient, the physician must consider the following points:

1. *What is the clinical problem that needs to be rectified or prevented?*

   The physician must have a clear understanding of the clinical problem to be addressed by transfusion in order to 1) formulate the most reasonable therapeutic plan and 2) as important, communicate the rationale for the plan to the patient.

2. *Does this problem warrant correction or prevention?*

   Is the problem a laboratory abnormality or does it correlate with or indicate a physiologic disturbance? Are there any significant clinical manifestations of these disturbances, indicating that the patient is not successfully compensating for them? The physician must be able to explain why it is important to correct or prevent the clinical problem that the transfusion is intended to address.

3. *Is the correction of the problem a clinically reasonable goal?*

   Is there reason, based either on a rationale grounded in an understanding of physiology or in clinical studies, to suppose that transfusion will correct the clinical problem? If the clinical problem is the result of multiple factors, only one of which can be corrected by transfusion, is the transfusion-correctable factor significant enough to outweigh the other factors and improve the clinical situation? The physician must be able to explain why it is believed that transfusion will be helpful to the patient.

4. *Is there a way to assess the benefit anticipated from the transfusion?*

Since transfusion therapy is often empiric, it is necessary to define the endpoint so that the effectiveness of the transfusion can be assessed. How can the basis for this assessment be communicated to the patient? The patient must understand the anticipated effects of the transfusion, especially when the endpoints are subjective (eg, energy level, exercise tolerance, etc), in order to provide the feedback necessary to evaluate the effectiveness of the transfusion.

5. *What are the indications for transfusion?*

In order to properly understand the likely benefits of transfusion, the physician should be aware of local or national guidelines that have been developed to aid making decisions about transfusion therapy. These published resources include practice guidelines suggested by several professional organizations, conclusions reached by the National Institutes of Health (NIH) Consensus Development Conferences, and key articles in the literature. While it is beyond the scope of this chapter to discuss in depth the indications for component therapy, the section below and the references listed at the end of the chapter should be helpful.

Resource Materials on Transfusion Indications

The following materials are offered as a resource only, and are not intended to represent a practice standard. Physicians should use their own judgment in making decisions about transfusions.

Red Blood Cells

An NIH Consensus Conference has established some broad indications for perioperative red blood cell transfusion.[1] Although the conclusion of the conference was that "No single measure can replace good clinical judgment as the basis for decisions regarding perioperative transfusion," it was also suggested that patients with hemoglobin levels exceeding 10 g/dL rarely require transfusion, while those with hemoglobin levels less than 7 g/dL frequently do. Several professional organizations have also established guidelines for red blood cell transfusion.[2-4] In addition to these general guidelines, several discussions of the process of making the decision to transfuse red blood cells have been published.[5-7]

Although the benefits of red cell transfusion are not always addressed directly, they may be inferred from studies correlating mortality[8-12] or other less drastic outcome measures[13-17] with degree of anemia or the use of various transfusion triggers.

Platelets

Indications for platelet transfusion have also been addressed by an NIH Consensus Conference[18] as well as by professional organizations.[3,19,20] Of particular interest in the last several years has been a reassessment of the use of prophylactic platelet transfusions in thrombocytopenic patients with marrow failure.[21] In general, the traditionally accepted trigger level of 20,000 platelets/μL for prophylactic transfusion is being replaced with a level of 10,000 platelets/μL.[22-24] However, some experts challenge the utility of prophylactic platelet transfusion suggesting that platelets should be administered only therapeutically.[25,26] Appropriate use of platelets in other settings has been reviewed.[27,28] There is some information about the role of platelet transfusion in a variety of clinical situations, including surgery[29-33] and other invasive procedures,[34-36] cardiopulmonary bypass,[37,38] and massive transfusion.[39,40]

Fresh Frozen Plasma (FFP)

Guidelines for clinical situations in which the use of FFP is likely to be of benefit have been established by an NIH Consensus Conference[41] as well as by some professional organizations.[3,19,42] The role for FFP transfusion in a variety of clinical settings has been reviewed.[43,44] FFP has been used as replacement for deficiencies of specific clotting factors and regulatory proteins, including proteins C and S,[45] or of multiple clotting factors.[36,46-48] The use of FFP for patients with mild coagulation abnormalities is probably not warranted. The risk of bleeding appears to be very low when the prothrombin time and partial thromboplastin time are only mildly elevated (<1.5 times the control,[49-51]) although this information needs to be reexamined in light of a better understanding of the variable sensitivity of these assays. FFP is also effective in the treatment of thrombotic thrombocytopenic purpura[52,53] and hemolytic uremic syndrome[54] and in reversing the effects of warfarin in an emergency situation.[55] Its roles in the treatment of disseminated intravascular coagulation,[56] massive transfusion,[57-60] and bleeding associated with cardiopulmonary bypass[61,62] have been discussed but are less well-defined.

Cryoprecipitated Antihemophilic Factor (Cryoprecipitate)

The use of cryoprecipitate has attracted less interest than that of other components, but published guidelines do exist,[3,19] and its use has been reviewed.[63] The practice of using this component as a source of fibrinogen[64] and Factor XIII[65] is well-accepted. In addition, some surgeons use cryoprecipitate with thrombin to form a topical anticoagulant, fibrin sealant.[66] The role of cryoprecipitate in the treatment of bleeding in uremic patients is controversial.[67,68]

Discussing the Benefits of Transfusion with the Patient

Only after the physician has defined the goal for the transfusion can its benefits be discussed productively with the patient. In describing the anticipated benefits of transfusion, the physician must be able to answer the following questions for the patient:

1. *What is the problem that the transfusion will correct or prevent?*

In making a risk/benefit assessment, each patient must weigh the gravity of the clinical problem, and its importance to him or her, against the risks of transfusion. Although the clinician may have an opinion about the clinical significance of the problem, the patient may view it in a different light, depending on the necessities and goals of his or her life.

2. *What is the rationale for the transfusion?*

   As part of an understanding of the potential benefit of a transfusion, the patient must have an appreciation for the likelihood that the desired outcome can be achieved. Part of that appreciation includes understanding the basis for the anticipated effect of the transfusions: Is the rationale for transfusion based on speculation, well-understood physiologic mechanisms, or the results of clinical trials? The patient must be able to factor the degree of certainty of achieving the desired result into the risk/benefit equation.

3. *What is the anticipated or desired effect of the transfusion?*

   The patient must understand what benefits are likely to be received from transfusion. What should the patient look for or expect after the transfusion? The type or magnitude of the benefit may color the willingness of the patient to assume risk. Patients need to assess for themselves whether the anticipated benefit is important to them or whether it will have a significant effect on the way they live.

Conclusion

The discussion of the benefits of transfusion beyond a description of the changes in certain laboratory values is not a trivial task. The physician wishing to give a patient the best information possible about the anticipated benefits of transfusion must first have very clear clinical objectives in mind. The definition of these objectives forms the basis on which the physician can describe the benefits that might result from transfusion. Following this successful communication, the patient can fairly balance the benefits of the transfusion against the risks, an assessment that lies at the heart of the process of informed consent.

References

1. NIH Consensus Development Conference. Perioperative red cell transfusion. JAMA 1992;260:2700-3.
2. American College of Physicians. Practice strategies for elective red blood cell transfusion. Ann Intern Med 1992;116: 403-6.
3. Stehling L, Luban NLC, Anderson KC, et al. Guidelines for blood utilization review. Transfusion 1994;34:438-48.
4. American Society of Anesthesiologists. Practice guidelines for blood transfusion. Anesthesiology 1996;84:732-47.
5. Welch HG, Meehan KR, Goodnough LT. Prudent strategies for elective red blood cell transfusion. Ann Intern Med 1992; 116:393-402.
6. Stehling J, Simon TL. The red cell transfusion trigger. Physiology and clinical studies. Arch Pathol Lab Med. 1994;118: 429-34.
7. Stowell CP. When to pull the trigger. Making the decision to transfuse red blood cells. Lab Med 1995;26:55-62.
8. Alexiu O, Mircea N, Balaban M, Furtunescu B. Gastrointestinal hemorrhage from peptic ulcer. An evaluation of bloodless transfusion and early surgery. Anaesthesia 1975;30:609-15.
9. Carson JL, Spence RK, Poses RM, Bonavita G. Severity of anaemia and operative mortality and morbidity. Lancet 1988;1:727-9.
10. Spence RK, Constabile JP, Young GS, et al. Is hemoglobin level alone a reliable predictor of outcome in the severely anemic surgical patient? Am Surg 1992;2:92-5.
11. Gould SA, Rosen AL, Sehgal LR, et al. Fluosol-DA as a red cell substitute in acute anemia. N Engl J Med 1986;314: 1953-6.
12. Kitchens CS. Are transfusions overrated? Surgical outcome of Jehovah's Witnesses. Am J Med 1993;94:117-19.

13. Kim DM, Brecher ME, Estes TJ, Morrey BF. Relationship of hemoglobin and duration of hospitalization after total hip arthroplasty: Implications for the transfusion target. Mayo Clin Proc 1993;68:37-41.
14. Johnson RG, Thurer RL, Kruskall MS, et al. Comparison of two transfusion strategies after elective operations for myocardial revascularization. J Thorac Cardiovasc Surg 1992; 104:307-14.
15. Lilleassen P, Stokke O. Moderate and extreme hemodilution in open-heart surgery: Fluid balance and acid-base studies. Ann Thorac Surg 1978;25:127-33.
16. Kawaguchi A, Bergsland J, Subramanian S. Total bloodless open heart surgery in the pediatric age group. Circulation 1984;70(Suppl 1):30-4.
17. Hébert PC, Wells G, Marshall J, et al. Transfusion requirements in critical care: A pilot study. JAMA 1995;273:1439-44.
18. NIH Consensus Development Conference. Platelet transfusion therapy. JAMA 1987;257:1777-80.
19. Fresh-Frozen Plasma, Cryoprecipitate, and Platelets Administration Practice Guidelines Development Task Force of the College of American Pathologists. Practice parameter for the use of fresh-frozen plasma, cryoprecipitate, and platelets. JAMA 1994;271:777-81.
20. British Committee for Standards in Haematology. Guidelines for platelet transfusions. Transfus Med 1992;2:311-28.
21. Beutler E. Platelet transfusions: The 20,000/μL trigger. Blood 1993;81:1411-3.
22. Gmür J, Burger J, Schanz U, et al. Safety of stringent prophylactic transfusion policy for patients with acute leukaemia. Lancet 1991;338:1223-6.
23. Heckman K, Weiner GJ, Strauss RG, et al. Randomized evaluation of optimal platelet count for prophylactic platelet transfusions in patients undergoing induction therapy for acute leukemia (abstract). Blood 1993;82(Suppl 1):192a.
24. Aderka D, Praff G, Santo, et al. Bleeding due to thrombocytopenia in acute leukemia and reevaluation of the prophylac-

tic platelet transfusion policy. Am J Med Sci 1986;291:147-51.

25. Soloman J, Bofenkamp T, Fahey JL, et al. Platelet prophylaxis in acute non-lymphoblastic leukemia (letter). Lancet 1978;1: 267.

26. Murphy S, Litwin S, Herring LM, et al. Indications for platelet transfusion in children with acute leukemia. Am J Hematol 1982;12:347-56.

27. Simpson MB. Platelet transfusion in selected clinical situations. In: Smith DM, Summers SH, eds. Platelets. Arlington, VA: American Association of Blood Banks. 1988:129-65.

28. Rintels PB, Kenney RM, Crowley JP. Therapeutic support of the patient with thrombocytopenia. Hematol Oncol Clin North Am. 1994;8:1131-57.

29. Bishop JF, Schiffer CA, Aisner J. Surgery in leukemia: A review of 167 operations in thrombocytopenic patients. Am J Hematol 1987;14:363-9.

30. Bjoernsson S, Yates J, Mittelman A, et al. Major surgery in acute leukemia. Cancer 1974;34:1272-5.

31. Rasmussen BL, Freeman JS. Major surgery in leukemia. Am J Surg 1975;130:647-51.

32. Hay A, Olsen KR, Nicholson DH. Bleeding complication in thrombocytopenic patients undergoing ophthalmic surgery. Am J Ophthalmol 1990;109:482-3.

33. Bergin JJ, Zuck TF, Miller RE. Compelling splenectomy in medically compromised patients. Ann Surg 1973;178:761-8.

34. Losowsky MS, Walker BE. Liver biopsy and splenoportography in patients with thrombocytopenia. Gastroenterology 1968;54:241-5.

35. Rasmus KT, Rotman RL, Dotelko DM, et al. Unrecognized thrombocytopenia and regional anesthesia in parturients: A retrospective review. Obstet Gynecol 1989;73:943.

36. McVay PA, Toy PTCY. Lack of increased bleeding after paracentesis and thoracentesis in patients with mild coagulation abnormalities. Transfusion 1991;31:164-71.

37. Goodnough LT, Johnston MFM, Ramsey G, et al. Guidelines for transfusion support in patients undergoing coronary artery bypass grafting. Ann Thorac Surg 1990;50:675-83.
38. Simpson MB. Prospective-concurrent audits and medical consultation for platelet transfusion. Transfusion 1987;27:192-5.
39. Ciavarella D, Reed RL, Counts RB, et al. Clotting factor levels and the risk of diffuse microvascular bleeding in the massively transfused patient. Br J Haematol 1987;67:365-8.
40. Reed RL II, Heimbach DM, Counts RB, et al. Prophylactic platelet administration during massive transfusion. A prospective, randomized, double-blind clinical study. Ann Surg 1986; 203:40-8.
41. NIH Consensus Development Conference. Fresh frozen plasma: Indications and risks. JAMA 1985;253:551-3.
42. British Committee for Standards in Haematology. Guidelines for fresh frozen plasma. Transfus Med 1992;2:57-63.
43. Braunstein AH, Oberman HA. Transfusion of plasma components. Transfusion 1984;24:281-6.
44. Humphries JE. Transfusion therapy in acquired coagulopathies. Hematol Oncol Clin North Am 1994;8:1181-201.
45. Comp PC, Esmon CT. Recurrent venous thrombosis in patients with a partial deficiency of protein S. N Engl J Med 1984;311:1525-8.
46. Davenport RD. Predicting postprocedure bleeding in liver disease. Hepatology 1992;15:735-7.
47. Gazzard BG, Henderson IM, Williams R. The use of fresh frozen plasma or a concentrate of Factor IX as replacement therapy before liver biopsy. Gut 1975;16:621-5.
48. Manucci PM, Franchi F, Dioguardi N. Correction of abnormal coagulation in chronic liver disease by combined use of fresh frozen plasma and prothrombin complex concentrates. Lancet 1976;2:542-5.
49. Hull R, Hirsh J, Jay R, et al. Different intensities of oral anticoagulant therapy in the treatment of proximal vein thrombosis. N Engl J Med 1982;307:1676-82.

50. Littman JK, Brodman HR. Surgery in the presence of the therapeutic effect of dicumarol. Surg Gynecol Obstet 1955; 101:709-14.
51. Rustad H, Myhre E. Surgery during anticoagulant treatment: The risk of increased bleeding in patients on oral anticoagulant treatment. Acta Med Scand 1963;173:115-9.
52. Bell WR, Braine HG, Ness PM, Kickler TS. Improved survival in thrombotic thrombocytopenic purpura-hemolytic uremic syndrome: Clinical experience with 108 patients. N Engl J Med 1991;325:398-403 [comment in N Engl J Med 1991; 325:426-8].
53. Rock GA, Shumak KH, Buskard NA, et al. Comparison of plasma exchange with plasma infusion in the treatment of thrombotic thrombocytopenic purpura. N Engl J Med 1991; 325:393-7.
54. Cattran DC. Adult hemolytic-uremic syndrome: Successful treatment with plasmapheresis. Am J Kidney Dis 1984;3: 275-9.
55. Fredriksson K, Norving B, Strömblad LG. Emergency reversal of anticoagulation after intracerebral hemorrhage. Stroke 1992;23:972-7.
56. Marder, VJ, Feinstein DJ, Francis CW, Colman RW. Consumptive thrombohemorrhagic disorders. In: Colman RW, Hirsh J, Marder VJ, Salzman EW, eds. Hemostasis and thrombosis: Basic principles and clinical practice. 3rd ed. Philadelphia: JB Lippincott. 1994:1023.
57. Counts RB, Haisch C, Simon TL, et al. Hemostasis in massively transfused trauma patients. Ann Surg 1979;190:91-9.
58. Leslie SD, Toy PTCY. Laboratory hemostatic abnormalities in massively transfused patients given red blood cells and crystalloid. Am J Pathol 1991;96:770-3.
59. Reiner A, Kickler TS, Bell WR. How to administer massive transfusions effectively. Guidelines for selecting blood components and monitoring reactions. J Crit Illn 1987;2:15-24.
60. Waters AH, Boulton FE, Dawson D, et al. Guidelines for transfusion for massive blood loss. Clin Lab Haematol 1988; 10:265-73.

61. Martinowitz U, Goor DA, Ramot B, et al. Is transfusion of fresh plasma after cardiac operations indicated? J Thorac Cardiovasc Surg 1990;100:92-8.
62. Roy RC, Stafford MA, Hudspeth AS, et al. Failure of prophylaxis with fresh frozen plasma after cardiopulmonary bypass. Anesthesiology 1988;69:254-7.
63. Poon MC. Cryoprecipitate; uses and alternatives. Transfus Med Rev 1993;7:180-92.
64. Ness PM, Perkins HA. Cryoprecipitate as a reliable source of fibrinogen replacement. JAMA 1979;241:1690-1.
65. Kitchens CS, Newcomb TF. Factor XIII. Medicine 1979;58: 413-29.
66. Gibble JW, Ness PM. Fibrin glue: The perfect operative sealant? Transfusion 1990;30:741-7.
67. Janson PA, Jubelirer SJ, Weinstein MJ, Deykin D. Treatment of the bleeding tendency in uremia with cryoprecipitate. N Engl J Med 1980;303:1318-22.
68. Remuzzi G. Bleeding in renal failure. Lancet 1988;1:1205-8.

In: Stowell, CP, ed.
Informed Consent for Blood Transfusion
Bethesda, MD: American Association of Blood Banks, 1997

6

Alternatives to Transfusion of Allogeneic Blood Components

Linda A. Chambers, MD

A key element of informed consent is discussion of the alternatives to the planned treatment—in this case, allogeneic transfusion from the general blood supply. As with expected benefits and risks, the applicable alternatives differ among patients, and for the same patient at various points in his or her disease and treatment.

This chapter discusses alternatives to, and options in, allogeneic blood transfusion. Many of the approaches are routine and generally known to be effective and appropriate for most patients, while others are investigational, of unproven clinical benefit, or applicable to only a subset of patients. Some of the treatments are extremely safe, while others have important risks that must be weighed against the risks of allogeneic transfusion.

The discussion is divided into three sections: transfusion-related alternatives, nontransfusion alternatives and options in allogeneic transfusion that may decrease risk. This chapter is not intended to recommend or advise against any particular treatment or option, nor should it be inferred that a nontransfusion alternative is always better. Rather, this discussion and the summary in Table 6-1 can be used to remind those making treatment deci-

Linda A. Chambers, MD, Chief of Clinical Pathology and Medical Director, Transfusion Service, Children's Hospital, Columbus, Ohio

Table 6-1. Alternatives to Allogeneic Transfusion

I. Transfusion-Related Alternatives
  A. Autologous transfusion
    1. Donation for autologous transfusion prior to elective surgery
    2. Perioperative blood recovery
    3. Preoperative hemodilution
    4. Preoperative plasmapheresis or plateletpheresis
  B. Conservative transfusion decisions
    1. Hold to strict indications
    2. Avoid "cocktails," "recipes," and empiric transfusion
    3. Give only the number of components required to achieve goal

II. Nontransfusion Alternatives
  A. Pharmacologic
    1. Correct deficiencies that could have necessitated transfusion
      a. Recombinant erythropoietin
      b. Desmopressin
      c. Granulocyte colony-stimulating factor or granulocyte-monocyte colony-stimulating factor
      d. Thrombopoietin
      e. Steroids
      f. High-dose intravenous immune globulin
      g. Iron, B_{12}, and folate
      h. Vitamin K
    2. Prevent deficiencies that could have necessitated transfusion
      a. Aprotinin and other antifibrinolytics
      b. Choice of drugs unlikely to cause cytopenias (eg low-molecular-weight heparin and heparinoids)
      c. Iron, B_{12}, folate, and vitamin K
  B. Nonpharmacologic
    1. Prevent a deficiency that might have necessitated transfusion
      a. "Bloodless" surgical techniques
      b. Optimal medical or surgical management of conditions associated with bleeding

(continued)

Table 6-1. Alternatives to Allogeneic Transfusion
(continued)

    2. Crystalloid, colloid, or oxygen-transporting solutions for
        a. Volume support and treatment of hemorrhagic shock
        b. Fluid replacement in therapeutic plasmapheresis
        c. Priming of cardiopulmonary bypass circuit prime

III. Options in Allogeneic Transfusion That May Decrease Risk
    A. Inventory
        1. Assigned unit practices
        2. Committed donor
        3. Multicomponent donor
        4. Single-donor apheresis platelets
        5. Directed donation
    B. Component preparation
        1. Irradiation
        2. Leukocyte reduction
        3. Cytomegalovirus low-risk
        4. Short-storage or washed packed red cells
        5. Red cell antigen-matching
        6. Virus inactivation

sions for a particular patient of some of the options that might be considered further.

Transfusion-Related Alternatives to Receiving Allogeneic Blood

Autologous Transfusion

Blood donation for autologous transfusion prior to elective surgery is a proven, highly effective strategy to reduce or prevent allogeneic blood exposure in patients who are scheduled for a surgical procedure likely to require transfusion. Most, but not all, of the infectious and noninfectious risks of transfusion are avoided when the blood is the patient's own. The only risks unique to autologous transfusion are those of the donation itself, presurgical anemia and delaying surgery to permit donation. All must be considered in the risk/benefit assessment on an individual patient basis.[1]

Other forms of autologous transfusion exist for surgical blood support. Probably the most widely applicable is perioperative blood recovery and reinfusion. Intraoperative recovery is most effective during major surgeries such as open-heart, vascular, or orthopedic procedures. Postoperative recovery of surgical site drainage is advantageous only when the postoperative red cell loss is substantial (ie, in excess of 150-200 mL red cells). Recovered blood must be reinfused within 6 hours of collection to avoid septic reactions to the bacteria with which these collections are frequently contaminated. Equipment options include simple filtration devices and automated wash-concentrate systems.[2,3]

Preoperative hemodilution—collecting several units of patient blood and replacing the volume with crystalloid or colloid solutions to establish isovolemic anemia just before surgery begins—may reduce net red cell loss when the expected volume of intraoperative blood loss is high and when the degree of anemia established by hemodilution is significant.[4] In a related procedure, a patient's platelets or platelet-rich plasma can be collected just before the start of surgery, maintained outside the patient for the duration of the procedure, and reinfused back postoperatively. Preoperative apheresis has been advocated for some open-heart procedures in the belief that it protects the removed platelets and coagulation proteins from any deleterious effects of cardiopulmonary bypass. After receiving undamaged autologous platelets and plasma, the patient may have improved postoperative hemostasis without allogeneic transfusion exposure.[5]

Conservative Transfusion Decisions

If support cannot be maintained with the patient's own blood, a first step in considering allogeneic transfusion is to critically reconsider whether transfusion is required at all.

The adoption of strict and conservative indications for transfusion and acceptance of normovolemic anemia in the perioperative period can substantially reduce the surgical red cell requirement. Active peer review of transfusion decisions and careful documentation of transfusion rationale in the medical record are also helpful.[6,7]

"Cocktails," "recipes," and "preventive" transfusion should be avoided, since most well-designed studies of empiric and prophylactic transfusions verify lack of effectiveness.[8,9] Physicians should be expected to prescribe only the number of components required to achieve the transfusion therapeutic goal. Indeed, even a single-unit transfusion (traditionally discouraged in favor of either no transfusion or a two-unit transfusion) is indicated if one unit is what the patient needs for symptomatic relief.

Nontransfusion Alternatives

Pharmacologic

Some deficiencies that might otherwise have required transfusion replacement can be corrected pharmacologically. Of the ever-increasing repertoire of recombinant hematopoietic growth factors, erythropoietin has proven especially effective for patients with anemia secondary to renal failure or other patients with inappropriately low serum erythropoietin, such as a subset of patients receiving AZT, bone marrow transplant recipients, and premature neonates.[10,11]

Growth factors and cytokines other than erythropoietin have corresponding focused clinical applications. Granulocyte colony-stimulating factor and granulocyte-monocyte colony-stimulating factor have been used successfully to reverse treatment-induced neutropenia, treat sepsis, and correct neonatal isoimmune neutropenia.[12] Thrombopoietin for hypoproliferative thrombocytopenias holds great promise.[13] Although thrombopoietin is not yet available for clinical use, basic research confirms the existence of this hematopoietic growth factor and its effect on megakaryocyte precursors; clinical trials are in progress.

The synthetic vasopressin analogue, desmopressin (DDAVP), has the serendipitous effect of inducing release of Factor VIII and von Willebrand factor (vWF), resulting in a twofold to fivefold increase in levels for several hours. DDAVP can be used to treat bleeding, or before minor invasive procedures, in patients with most subtypes of von Willebrand's disease or mild Factor VIII deficiency.[14] Probably because of its effect on vWF and the dependence of platelet-endothelial adherence on vWF activity, DDAVP also shortens the bleeding time and may help control clinical bleeding in patients with uremia and some other types of acquired or congenital disorders of platelet function.[15]

Additional pharmacologic treatments may correct cytopenias and coagulopathies that would otherwise require blood transfusion.[16-18] Steroids and high-dose intravenous immune globulin are used in the treatment of idiopathic thrombocytopenic purpura; iron, B_{12}, and folate are used for deficiency-related anemias; intravenous immune globulin is used for neonatal isoimmune thrombocytopenia and hemolytic disease of the newborn; and vitamin K is used to reverse warfarin anticoagulation.

In other clinical circumstances, pharmacologic agents may be used not only to correct, but also to prevent, deficiencies that might have required transfusion. Aprotinin and related antifibrinolytics have been reported to lower blood loss and red cell transfusion requirements substantially in patients in a high fibrinolytic state such as that occurring after open-heart surgery.[19,20] Aprotinin has the additional benefits of protecting platelet function and reducing coagulation protein activation during cardiopulmonary bypass. These effects improve postoperative coagulation, thereby lowering both chest tube red cell loss and the clinical need for non-red-cell-component transfusion.[21,22]

Avoiding drugs that are likely to cause thrombocytopenia (eg, low-molecular-weight heparin and heparinoids); ensuring adequate iron, B_{12}, and folate supplementation for infants and pregnant women; and prescribing vitamin K supplementation for neonates and patients with liver disease may reduce the likelihood of transfusion of platelets, red cells, and fresh frozen plasma (FFP), respectively.

Nonpharmacologic

Both allogeneic and autologous transfusions can be minimized or avoided using techniques, referred to collectively as "blood conservation" in the surgical setting, that are intended to minimize blood loss. Adoption of "bloodless" surgical techniques and optimal medical or surgical management of conditions associated with bleeding, such as placenta previa and esophageal varices can lower the overall rate of transfusion of any sort (including preoperatively donated autologous blood, and, perioperative recovered autologous and allogeneic blood). Systematic use of nonblood alternatives such as crystalloid, colloid, or oxygen-transporting solutions for such needs as volume support, treatment for hemorrhagic shock, fluid replacement in therapeutic plasmapheresis and priming of the cardiopulmonary bypass circuit, minimize allogeneic transfusion rates and donor exposures in these settings.

Options in Allogeneic Transfusion that May Decrease Risk

Inventory

When transfusion is unavoidable and autologous components are not available, the risk of allogeneic transfusion support can be lowered by use of special inventory programs. Limiting the total number of required donor exposures may lower the cumulative infectious risk as well as incidence of noninfectious complications such as red cell antibody formation. For neonates and infants, this can be accomplished easily by assigning units to one or several patients. Preparing multiple small-volume aliquot transfusions from one donor unit for a given neonate can reduce donor exposures by more than half.[23] For larger children and adult patients, one donor may make a series of donations for a given chronic transfusion recipient (committed donor) or donate two or more components to be used by the same patient (multicomponent donor).[24] Multicomponent donation might be planned at the time of donation or orchestrated in the transfusion service when, for example,

FFP and red cells of the same component number are used to prepare a unit of reconstituted whole blood. Use of single-donor apheresis platelets in lieu of pooled concentrates decreases donor exposures as well as the likelihood of formation of platelet-reactive (HLA or other) antibodies.[25] This option, however, has limited availability and may be less useful for patients who are already receiving leukocyte-reduced components to lower the rate of HLA antibody formation. Furthermore, because the known transfusion infection risks are now well below 1/10,000 with current donor selection and testing practices (see chapter 3), the difference in infection risk between, for example, 10 and 20 donor exposures may not be medically significant.*

Directed donation is a transfusion option when the patient or a designee recruits the donors of needed blood components. There is no generally accepted evidence of any increased safety with directed donation.[26] However, it may provide an opportunity to establish a committed donor or multicomponent donor relationship as described above, which does reduce total donor exposures.

Component Preparation

Among other options in allogeneic transfusion that affect the risk is the proper use of specially processed or selected components—irradiated cellular components to prevent transfusion graft-vs-host disease; leukocyte-reduced components to prevent febrile, nonhemolytic transfusion reactions or to delay HLA antibody formation; cytomegalovirus (CMV) low-risk components for CMV-negative recipients; or short-storage or washed red cells for high-volume transfusion.[27-29] Transfusion services with planned

---

* If the risk of an infection is 1/10,000 (0.0001) per donor exposure, then infection does not occur with 9999/10,000 (0.9999) donor exposures. When a patient receives 20 donor exposures, the probability of avoiding infection is $(0.9999)^{20}$ or 0.9980 (998/1000 receive no infection, 2/1000 become infected). If, through a limited-donor program, the donor exposures are reduced to 10, the probability of avoiding infection increases only to 0.9999^{10} or 0.9990 (999/1000 receive no infection, 1/1000 becomes infected). Complication rates of 1/1000 or 2/1000 are sufficiently low that the difference would not be apparent at the transfusion volumes of a typical hospital. (Remember, a predicted probability of 1/1000 *on average* does not mean there will be any cases at all at a specific hospital tracking 1000 or 2000 or even 3000 donor exposures.)

systems for identifying patients requiring special components are most effective in ensuring these preventive interventions.

Total or partial red cell antigen matching lowers the risk of red cell antibody formation in recipients of chronic repeated red cell transfusions.[30] This strategy may be particularly valuable for patients at high risk for forming multiple antibodies because of patient-donor pool antigen distribution differences and for patients who have lifelong, sometimes intense red cell transfusion requirements. Patients with sickle cell disease or thalassemia major fit both criteria.

Other than for blood derivatives such as Factor VIII concentrates, virus inactivation methods for transfusion components, such as pasteurization and solvent-detergent treatment, remain under development. Additionally, except for derivatives manufactured from pools of the blood of thousands of donors, any reduction in the already low risk of residual infection may not be medically important until, and unless, all types of components are inactivated.

Conclusions

Obtaining informed consent should include a discussion of alternatives to, and within, the planned therapy. In the case of transfusion, alternatives involve such diverse considerations as nontransfusion treatments, preventive strategies, donor options, special inventory management programs, and optimal medical decision-making. Each option presents its own predicted efficacy and risk that must be factored into the complicated assessment of the best medical advice for a particular patient at a specific point in treatment.

References

1. Chambers LA, Kruskall MS. Preoperative autologous blood donation. Transfus Med Rev 1990;4:35-46.

2. Dzik WH, Sherburne B. Intraoperative blood salvage: Medical controversies. Transfus Med Rev 1990;4:208-35.
3. Eng J, Kay PH, Murday AG, et al. Postoperative autologous transfusion in cardiac surgery. A prospective, randomised study. Eur J Cardiothorac Surg 1990;4:595-600.
4. Ness PM, Bourke DL, Walsh PC. A randomized trial of perioperative hemodilution versus transfusion of preoperative deposited autologous blood in elective surgery. Transfusion 1991;31:226-30.
5. Davies GG, Wells DG, Mabee TM, et al. Platelet-leukocyte plasmapheresis attenuates the deleterious effects of cardiopulmonary bypass. Ann Thorac Surg 1992;53:274-7.
6. Stehling L, Luban NLC, Anderson KC, et al. Guidelines for blood utilization review. Transfusion 1994;34:438-48.
7. Silberstein LE, Kruskall MS, Stehling LC, et al. Strategies for the review of transfusion practices. JAMA 1989;262:1993-7.
8. Simon TL, Alk BF, Murphy W. Controlled trial of routine administration of platelet concentrates in cardiopulmonary bypass surgery. Ann Thorac Surg 1984;37:359-64.
9. Martin DJ, Lucas CE, Ledgerwood AM, et al. Fresh frozen plasma supplement to massive red blood cell transfusion. Ann Surg 1985;202:505-11.
10. Maier RF, Obladen M, Scigalla P, et al. The effect of epoetin beta on the need for transfusion in very-low-birth-weight infants. N Engl J Med 1994;330:1173-8.
11. Eschbach JW, Abdulhadi MH, Browne JK, et al. Recombinant human erythropoietin in anemia patients with end-stage renal disease. Ann Intern Med 1989;111:992-1000.
12. Gabrilove J. The development of granulocyte colony-stimulating factor in its various clinical applications. Blood 1992;80:1382-5.
13. Schick BP. Hope for treatment of thrombocytopenia. N Engl J Med 1994;331:875-6.
14. Manucci PM. Desmopressin: A nontransfusional form of treatment for congenital and acquired bleeding disorders. Blood 1988;72:1449-55.

15. Schulman S. DDAVP—the multipotent drug in patients with coagulopathies. Transfus Med Rev 1991;5:132-44.
16. MacIntyre EA, Linch DC, Macey MG, et al. Successful response to intravenous immunoglobulin in autoimmune haemolytic anemia. Br J Haematol 1985;60:387-8.
17. Bussel JB, Berkowitz RL, McFarland JG, et al. Antenatal treatment of neonatal alloimmune thrombocytopenia. N Engl J Med 1988;319:1374-8.
18. Rubo J, Albrecht K, Lasch P, et al. High-dose intravenous immune globulin therapy for hyperbilirubinemia caused by Rh hemolytic disease. J Pediatr 1992;121:93-7.
19. DelRossi AJ, Cernaianu AC, Botros S, et al. Prophylactic treatment of postperfusion bleeding using EACA. Chest 1989;96:27-30.
20. Suarez M, Sangro B, Herrero JI, et al. Effectiveness of aprotinin in orthotopic liver transplantation. Semin Thromb Hemost 1993;19:292-6.
21. VanOeveren W, Harder MP, Roozendaal KJ, et al. Aprotinin protects platelets against the initial effect of cardiopulmonary bypass. J Thorac Cardiovasc Surg 1990;99:788-97.
22. VanOeveren W, Jansen NJ, Bidstrup BP, et al. Effects of aprotinin on hemostasis mechanisms during cardiopulmonary bypass. Ann Thorac Surg 1987;44:640-5.
23. Cook S, Gunter J, Wissel M. Effective use of a strategy using assigned red cell units to limit donor exposure for neonatal patients. Transfusion 1993;33:379-83.
24. Strauss RG, Wieland MR, Randels MJ, et al. Feasibility and success of a single-donor red cell program for pediatric elective surgery patients. Transfusion 1992;32:747-9.
25. Sintnicolaas K, Sizoo W, Haije WG, et al. Delayed alloimmunization by random single donor platelet transfusion. Lancet 1981;1(8223):750-4.
26. Cordell RR, Yalon VA, Cagahn-Haskell C, et al. Experience with 11,916 designated donors. Transfusion 1986;26:484-6.
27. Anderson KC, Goodnough LT, Sayers M, et al. Variation in blood component irradiation practice: Implications for pre-

vention of transfusion-associated graft-versus-host disease. Blood 1991;77:2096-102.

28. Ciavarella D. Introduction: Leukocyte-depleted blood products. Transfus Med Rev 1990;4:1-2.

29. Kickler TS. The challenge of platelet alloimmunization: management and prevention. Transfus Med Rev 1990;4:8-18.

30. Tahhan HR, Holbrook CT, Braddy LR, et al. Antigen-matched donor blood in the transfusion management of patients with sickle cell disease. Transfusion 1994;34:562-9.

In: Stowell, CP, ed.
Informed Consent for Blood Transfusion
Bethesda, MD: American Association of Blood Banks, 1997

7

Informed Consent Policies and Procedures

Thomas A. Lane, MD; Irena Sniecinski, MD; and Christopher P. Stowell, MD, PhD

Implementation of informed consent for blood transfusion in an institution requires two key elements: an institutional policy on informed consent and procedures describing how the policy is to be effected. For institutions interested in developing a position regarding informed consent, this chapter addresses both elements. It describes the important components of an informed consent policy for transfusion and the resources and personnel who should be part of the development process. The chapter also contains a discussion of the components included in procedures that guide personnel carrying out the institutional policy.

Examples of alternative methods for implementing informed consent policies and procedures are included at the end of the chapter. The American Association of Blood Banks does not require informed consent for blood transfusion,[1] nor does it specifically endorse any of the examples provided. The examples are included solely to demonstrate different approaches; each

Thomas A. Lane, MD, Medical Director, Transfusion Services, School of Medicine, University of California at San Diego, La Jolla, California; Irena Sniecinski, MD, Director, Transfusion Medicine, Department of Clinical Pathology, City of Hope Medical Center, Duarte, California; and Christopher P. Stowell, MD, PhD, Director, Blood Transfusion Service, Massachusetts General Hospital and Department of Pathology, Harvard Medical School, Boston, Massachusetts

institution should develop its own policies and procedures, as dictated by its unique situation.

Developing a Policy

The need for a policy that specifically addresses consent for transfusion should first be discussed by whatever executive committee/body of the organization develops informed consent for other situations. The decision to obtain informed consent specifically for transfusion and the determination of the manner in which that consent is obtained should be considered in the context of the institution's approach to informed consent in general.

Once an institution decides that, indeed, a policy is needed, pertinent data should be gathered. The institution should determine if there are local or state regulatory statutes and case law that affect some aspects of informed consent for transfusion. Likewise, information from professional organizations should be collected and compared.[2-4] Institutions should consider prevailing medical practice to ensure that any proposed policies meet or exceed that standard.

With available resources in hand, the executive committee should broaden the discussion group to include transfusion medicine experts, physicians and nurses involved in transfusion therapy, and the hospital legal counsel. The involvement of a patient care advocate and an ethicist is highly desirable. It may be appropriate for members of the hospital transfusion committee to provide input, either through a recommendation prepared after a discussion of the issues from their perspective or through a representative included in the discussion group. If the institution's general patient population includes Jehovah's Witnesses, then either a representative of those patients or a person within the institution who is familiar with their beliefs may be a helpful participant.

Once the discussion group defines an institutional policy for informed consent for transfusion, an individual or group within the institution should be designated to draft the procedures that will direct all personnel in carrying out the policy. The individuals who are responsible for other transfusion procedures should work out the details of the procedure for obtaining and documenting informed consent.

Components of a Policy on Informed Consent for Blood Transfusion

Although each institution should formulate its own policy in the context of its own situation, several basic components are shared by most policies. The institutional policy statement on informed consent for blood transfusion should include at a minimum the following components.

The Elements of Informed Consent

The policy should broadly define what is meant by informed consent. Chapter 1 discusses generally accepted elements of informed consent.

The Purpose of Obtaining Informed Consent

The purpose should in some way convey the intent that patients should have the information and the ability (to the fullest extent possible) to make an informed choice with regard to the available alternatives for treatment.

The Applicability of Informed Consent

The policy should define the situations in which informed consent for blood transfusion should be obtained. In general, virtually all transfusions should be covered. However, emergency situations in which it may be impractical or dangerous to obtain informed consent should represent an exception. The policy should define these exceptional situations in which consent need not be obtained. The institution should also define the blood components and derivatives for the transfusion of which informed consent should be obtained.

Who May Consent

The policy should delineate who may provide informed consent. Provisions should be made for 1) patients who are physically or mentally incompetent to give consent and 2) minors, including emancipated minors (see Chapter 2). The policy should define under which circumstances reliance on a surrogate decision-maker is acceptable.

The Frequency of Obtaining Informed Consent

Depending on applicable law (see Chapter 2), the policy should provide guidelines regarding the frequency with which it is necessary to repeat the process of obtaining informed consent. An institution may elect to obtain informed consent before each and every transfusion. Alternatively, an institution may elect to define a period (such as a single hospital stay) or a course of care for which a single informed consent event shall apply.

If consent is to be applied to more than one transfusion episode, the institution should establish guidelines defining the period or course of care. If informed consent is given for a period or course of care, it must be obtained again if the risks, benefits, or alternatives originally discussed with the patient are altered by changes in transfusion therapy (eg, introduction of a component or derivative treated to reduce virus transmission) or the patient's condition (eg, development of renal failure or congestive heart failure).

The Personnel Obtaining Informed Consent

In accordance with applicable law (see Chapter 2), the policy should define who has the responsibility for obtaining and documenting informed consent. Most often, the physician who is making the decision about transfusion therapy is the individual who obtains and documents the informed consent of a patient. In a complex health-care environment, however, it is possible that different individuals may be involved in the process of educating the patient, answering patient questions, discussing alternatives to allogeneic transfusion, documenting that consent has been obtained, and verifying that the consent has been documented before transfusion.

In general, responsibility remains with the physician; however, the reader is cautioned to comply with applicable laws and regulations.

Information Provided to the Patient

The nature of the information provided to the patient is generally determined by the physician obtaining the consent. The physician should be knowledgeable about the risks, benefits, and alternatives of the proposed therapy. The institution does not ordinarily determine the content or extent of this information. However, in some circumstances, particularly when state law mandates that certain information shall be provided to patients (eg, California), the institution may elect to specify that this required information be conveyed during the informed consent process. The institution may choose to provide printed material describing the risks, benefits, and alternatives to allogeneic transfusion therapy. For patients undergoing common procedures, the information provided to patients should include the likelihood of transfusion.

The discussion of informed consent should reflect the particular risks and benefits presented by the proposed transfusion therapy *for the individual patient*, which may depend on the patient's medical condition. The discussion must be tailored to the patient's educational level and ability not only to comprehend the language in which the discussion takes place, but also to respond in that language. Those risks that are pertinent to the patient must be described. Depending on the applicable legal standard (see Chapter 2), the patient should be provided with the information that a reasonable person would require to make an informed decision to accept or reject the proposed transfusion therapy.

Internal Compliance

The policy should describe who is responsible for ensuring compliance with the policy. The institution may assign responsibility to the Transfusion Committee, the Department of Nursing, the Quality Assurance Unit, or some other group. The policy should also specify the manner in which compliance is reviewed by medical staff.

Compliance with Regulations

The policy should include appropriate references to requirements of applicable local, state, and federal agencies that set standards for or regulate institutional operations.

Other Guidelines

The institution may find it helpful to refer to voluntary guidelines established by professional organizations such as the Joint Commission on Accreditation of Healthcare Organizations. The policy should also refer to other applicable institutional policies such as general policies on informed consent, guidelines on patients' rights, blood transfusion policies, and policies regarding Jehovah's Witnesses.

Documentation

The policy should include standard institutional policy information such as dates of implementation and review, approval of authorized individual, a statement on the applicability to various institutional divisions or locations, and a record of prior versions of the policy.

Examples

As noted above, these elements are only the most basic requirements shared by most policies on informed consent for transfusion. Organizations should strive to exceed these minimums and create policies that are appropriate for their unique environment.

Additionally, the content of an institutional informed consent policy should vary to comply with local and state law. The format used will depend on the needs and practices of each individual institution.

Two different approaches to a policy on informed consent for transfusion are shown in Appendix 7-1 and 7-2. These examples are included for illustration only; their inclusion does not constitute the endorsement of the American Association of Blood Banks. In Appendix 7-1, the institution has established a specific and separate policy for informed consent for transfusion. One advantage of this approach is that transfusion-specific issues can be addressed in detail. In addition, someone unfamiliar with the specific policy of informed consent for transfusion in that institution can find the relevant information in a succinct form.

In Appendix 7-2, informed consent for transfusion is included within the context of the institution's general informed consent policy. One advantage of this approach is that some degree of consistency is ensured for the informed consent obtained under various circumstances. In addition, some degree of redundancy among similar policies is eliminated.

Components of Procedures for Informed Consent for Blood Transfusion

Once policies for informed consent for transfusion have been established, procedures should be written that delineate the specific steps taken by institutional personnel to obtain and document informed consent. As for policies, each institution should create its own written procedures. However, several basic elements are common to such procedures.

Procedure Information and Approvals

As with any other procedure, the informed consent procedure should include the title of the procedure, the names and titles of the persons who are responsible for writing and approving the procedure, and the dates of approval and implementation.

Relevant Policies

The procedure should cross-reference relevant general policies and present them in summary fashion. In addition, other relevant policies about blood transfusion should be summarized.

Personnel

The procedure should specify who is permitted to obtain and document informed consent. Ordinarily, the physician making the decision about transfusion therapy bears the responsibility for obtaining consent; however, this may not always be the case. Persons responsible for each step in the process (eg, document handling, compliance, verification that consent has been obtained) should be clearly identified.

Scope of the Procedure

If there are procedural variations in different settings (eg, outpatient vs inpatient), the procedure should define the clinical areas to which each step of the procedure applies.

Applicability

If not defined in the informed consent policy, the circumstances under which informed consent should be obtained and from whom it may be obtained must be included in the procedure.

Required Elements

If not otherwise specified by the informed consent policy, the institution may elect to specify in the procedure what information is to be conveyed to the patient during the informed consent process.

Method for Obtaining Informed Consent

This is the heart of the procedure, where specific instructions are provided for the step-by-step process by which informed consent is obtained and documented. For example, there may be separate and somewhat different procedures for inpatients and outpatients. Obviously, the simple presentation of written information to a patient is insufficient. In addition to specific instructions for each step in the process, the procedure should specify the individual responsible for accomplishing each of the steps.

The procedure should also provide identification of the forms required, as well as how and by whom they are to be completed and recorded. Samples of correctly completed forms should be included with the procedure.

Documentation and Data Management

The procedure must also describe the method used to retain information pertaining to the record of either the patient's informed consent or the patient's rejection of the transfusion procedure. If this documentation includes a form signed by the patient and the caregiver providing the information and answering the patient's questions, the procedure must specify where this form is retained. If retention of this information is electronic, the procedure should describe a means to access the information.

Pretransfusion Verification

The procedure should specify that the transfusionist verifies documentation of informed consent before the actual transfusion takes place. Verification can be made by checking the appropriate box on a requisition form, writing a brief note in the chart, or making an electronic entry into the computer record.

Quality Assurance and Medical Staff Review

The procedure should define the nature and extent of the medical staff review for compliance with institutional policy on informed consent. The method should define goals of the review and the criteria for adequate performance. It should specify the frequency of review and/or the sample size, how and by whom the review is to be accomplished, and the method of reporting the results of the review to the medical staff.

Examples of indicators that reviewers might use include: 1) Is informed consent obtained on all indicated patients? 2) Are all elements of informed consent accomplished? 3) Is informed consent obtained in a timely fashion? 4) Is documentation up-to-date and available?

Examples

Two examples of informed consent procedures are shown in Appendix 7-3 and Appendix 7-4. Appendix 7-3 shows an independent informed consent procedure. Such a procedure has the advantage of specific, clear steps that facilitate an understanding of the procedure in this institution. Note that this institution also uses checklists to help physicians and nurses to verify that all of the various elements of the informed consent process have been accomplished. In addition, a copy of the information that the institution provides to transfusion candidates is provided.

In Appendix 7-4, another approach is illustrated. In this procedure, the steps for verifying informed consent are embedded in the transfusion procedure. This approach has the advantage of all relevant transfusion steps located together in a single procedure that more closely follows the workflow.

Conclusion

The distinction between a policy and a procedure is often a fine one. In some instances, policy statements may be quite detailed and take on some characteristics of procedures. In other cases, policies may be very broad and their intent may be clarified in the procedures manual.

In general, physician "procedures" are not as well-described as procedures for other personnel. It is not uncommon for an institution's policy statements to specify areas of physician responsibility without describing those areas in much detail. This is often the case with policies for informed consent for transfusion. An institutional policy may merely specify that a patient's physician is responsible for obtaining informed consent and define the circumstances in which consent must be obtained. There may be no step-by-step description of the physician's activity in this regard.

When a step-by-step description of informed consent is not specified in either the policies or procedures, the emphasis is on the outcomes: Has the patient been given adequate information to make an informed decision? Has the patient made a decision? Has the physician documented the interaction with the patient?

References

1. Informed consent for blood transfusion. Association Bulletin #94-3. Bethesda, MD: American Association of Blood Banks, September 1, 1994.
2. Comprehensive accreditation manual for hospitals. Oakbrook Terrace, IL: Joint Commission on Accreditation of Healthcare Organizations, 1995.
3. Meisel A, Kuczewski M. Legal and ethical myths about informed consent. Arch Intern Med 1990;156:2521-6.
4. Widmann FK. Informed consent for blood transfusion: Brief historical survey and summary of a conference. Transfusion 1990;30:460-70.

Appendix 7-1. Example of a Separate Policy for Informed Consent for Transfusion

INSTITUTION POLICY: INFORMED CONSENT FOR ADMINISTRATION OF

BLOOD OR BLOOD COMPONENTS

XYZ Institution, Anywhere, USA

Title and Abstract Page

Institution Policy: IP-123.1
Effective Date: 1/1/96 --- Revised 3/1/96 ---
Supercedes: IP-123.1; 1/1/95
For Policy Review on: 1/1/97
Institution Applicability: _x_ Medical Center A;   _x_ Medical Center B
                               _x_ Outpatient Surgicenter A;   _x_ HomeCare Program

Distribution: Institution Policy and Procedure Manual Distribution List

Re: IP-123.1

    This Policy and Procedure has been revised and reissued. Provided below is a summary.
To receive the full text of the instruction, pleas contact Institutional Administrative Services at x
1-1234

REFERENCES:

    1. State Health & Safety Code, Section 123, "The John Doe Blood Safety Act"
    2. JCAHO Accreditation Manual, Patient Rights
    3. JCAHO Accreditation Manual, Operative and Other Invasive Procedures
    4. State Association of Hospitals and Health Systems "Consent Manual"
    5. State Code of Regulations, Title 12, Licensing and Certification of Health Facilities
and Referral Agencies, Section 10101 - Patient Rights
    6. AABB Informed Consent Statement, 1996

ABSTRACT: This Policy and Procedure is designed to provide guidelines for informing the
patient of transfusion alternatives and risks and obtaining patient consent when the transfusion of
blood or blood components is required or anticipated. Patients have the right to make informed
decisions about their transfusion options if there is a reasonable possibility that the non-emergent
administration of blood or blood components may be necessary.

Signature, Director   Date
Institution Medical Centers
   and Clinics

XYZ Institution, Anywhere, USA

Institution Policy: IP-123.1
Effective Date: 1/1/96 --- Revised 3/1/96 ---
Supercedes: IP-123.1; 1/1/95
For Policy Review on: 1/1/97
Institution Applicability: _x_ Medical Center A;   _x_ Medical Center B
                               _x_ Outpatient Surgicenter A;   _x_ HomeCare Program

IP#:   123.1

TITLE: INFORMED CONSENT FOR ADMINISTRATION OF BLOOD OR BLOOD COMPONENTS

REGULATORY REFERENCES:

1. State Health & Safety Code, Section 123, "The John Doe Blood Safety Act"
2. JCAHO Accreditation Manual, Patient Rights
3. JCAHO Accreditation Manual, Operative and Other Invasive Procedures
4. State Association of Hospitals and Health Systems "Consent Manual"
5. State Code of Regulations, Title 12, Licensing and Certification of Health Facilities
and Referral Agencies, Section 10101 - Patient Rights
6. AABB Informed Consent Statement, 1996

RELATED INSTITUTIONAL POLICIES:

1. IP-111.1   Informed Consent
2. IP-234.1   Patient Rights
3. IP-345.1   Interpreter Services
4. IP-456.1   Reporting Reaction to Blood or Blood Components
5. IP-567.1   Emergency Requests for Blood

KEY WORDS: blood, blood components, blood products, autologous donation, directed donation, informed consent, transfusion options

I.   Purpose:

To set forth Institution guidelines for a) educating patients regarding transfusion options and alternatives, and b) for obtaining patient consent when there is a reasonable possibility that a transfusion of blood or blood components is required. This policy is

Institutional Policy # 123.1; 1/1/96; revised - 3/1/96

XYZ Institution, Anywhere, USA

Institution Policy: IP-123.1
Effective Date: 1/1/96 --- Revised 3/1/96 ---
Supercedes: IP-123.1; 1/1/95
For Policy Review on: 1/1/97
Institution Applicability: _x_ Medical Center A;   _x_ Medical Center B
                              _x_ Outpatient Surgicenter A;   . _x_ HomeCare Program

also meant to comply with the legal mandates of this State with regard to patient
education and offering transfusion options and alternatives.

II.   Definitions:

A. Informed Consent: A process whereby the physician informs the patient regarding
the nature of the treatment, the risk, complications, expected benefits of such treatment,
the alternatives to the recommended treatment, the likely results of no treatment, the
probability that the recommended treatment will be successful, and any additional
information the patient may need to make a reasonable decision regarding the
recommended treatment. The patient must have a reasonable opportunity to discuss any
questions, issues or concerns and to reach a decision to accept or reject the transfusion.

B. Consent Form: A document that verifies the patient's signature confirming that the
patient has discussed the treatment or procedure with the physician, understands the
information, and has given his or her informed consent to the physician.

C. Emergency Procedure: An emergency procedure is any diagnostic or therapeutic
procedure which, in the judgment of the attending physician, must be performed within a
time period defined by the institution, eg 24 hours, in order to avoid an adverse effect on
the patient's course or likelihood of recovery.

D. Blood and Blood Components: Blood and Blood Components are therapeutic agents
derived from human blood, which are designed to support blood oxygen carrying
capacity, hemostasis, or immune function, regardless of processing or purification.
Albumin and plasma protein fraction are exempt from this definition.

III.   Scope of Policy:

A. Patients have the right to make informed decisions about their transfusion options if
there is a reasonable possibility that the non-emergent administration of blood or blood
components may be necessary.

XYZ Institution, Anywhere, USA

Institution Policy: IP-123.1
Effective Date: 1/1/96 --- Revised 3/1/96 ---
Supercedes: IP-123.1; 1/1/95
For Policy Review on: 1/1/97
Institution Applicability: _x_ Medical Center A;   _x_ Medical Center B
                                _x_ Outpatient Surgicenter A;   , _x_ HomeCare Program

B. This policy shall not apply when medical contraindications of a life-threatening emergency exists. If it is determined that a procedure is urgently indicated and that time will not allow for the elements of this policy to be fulfilled, the physician shall write a brief explanatory not in the medical record.

C. Some patients, due to age, mental status, or other factors, may have surrogate decision makers, either family members, or those assigned by state authorities. This policy will apply to authorized surrogate decision makers (referred to as the "patient's representative), when applicable. (See IP-234.1 Patient Rights)

D. A list of invasive procedures in the Institution Transfusion Manual for Physicians (Attachment 1) should serve as a guideline to the Attending Physicians and Physicians in Training for blood ordering practices and the likelihood that there is a reasonable possibility of a blood product transfusion.

E. State law requires that, unless there is a life-threatening medical contraindication, physicians and surgeons shall allow adequate time prior to the procedure for predonation to occur, or for other transfusion options or alternatives. In general, this may require 3 to 15 days. The patient has the right to waive the adequate time for predonation, but should not be encouraged to do so.

F. For patients who require repeated blood and blood product transfusion for the same indication, Informed Consent for Administration of Blood and Blood Components may be considered to be in effect, unless revoked by the patient, for up to 12 months, or until new information, a new blood product, or new treatment becomes available which alters the risks and / or benefits as previously discussed with the patient, or a change in the patient's health status affects the risks and/or potential benefits of transfusion. In such cases, a new Informed Consent should be obtained and documented.

IV.   Procedures, Responsibilities, and Requirements:

A.   The physician or surgeon who first proposes to schedule a patient for an invasive procedure and who orders that a blood type and antibody screen or compatibility test be performed is responsible for discussing and documenting the patient's education and

XYZ Institution, Anywhere, USA

Institution Policy: IP-123.1
Effective Date: 1/1/96 --- Revised 3/1/96 ---
Supercedes: IP-123.1; 1/1/95
For Policy Review on: 1/1/97
Institution Applicability: _x_ Medical Center A;   _x_ Medical Center B
                                _x_ Outpatient Surgicenter A;   _x_ HomeCare Program

wishes regarding the possibility of blood or blood product administration. For any procedure that will require a blood type, with or without an antibody screen, or compatibility test the physician:

1. shall discuss the possibility of blood transfusion with the patient or representative, the risks and benefits of transfusion, the methods whereby blood transfusion may be avoided or minimized (if applicable), the positive and negative aspects of receiving homologous blood, predonating and receiving autologous blood and, as directed by our State Law, the positive and negative aspects of receiving directed and nondirected homologous blood from volunteer donors.

2. shall complete, sign, and provide the patient or representative with a blood transfusion information and consent form entitled "Patient Information & Consent - Transfusion Options and Alternatives" (Institution Form 123-456; Attachment 2).

3. shall ensure compliance with State Law, which requires that the patient or representative be given a copy of the "State Department of Health Services brochure entitled, "A Patient's Guide to Blood Transfusion" (Attachment 3). The "Transfusion Options..." form, along with the "Institution Universal Consent to Invasive Procedure" form (Attachment 4) are to be used together and the physician will ensure that both are administered and signed.

4. shall allow the patient adequate time prior to the procedure for autologous predonation of blood or blood components to occur, except in life-threatening emergencies, when medically contraindicated, or when the patient waives the right to allow adequate time for predonation. This information shall be documented by the patient via the "Transfusion Options...." form and by the physician via a detailed entry in the patient's medical record. Since it may require longer than 15 days to collect sufficient autologous blood, physicians should schedule patients for autologous blood donations at the earliest possible time after an invasive procedure date has been set. Blood can be stored in the liquid state for up to 42 days, and, if frozen, indefinitely.

5. shall, if the patient or representative refuses to permit blood transfusion, ensure that the "Refusal to Permit Blood Transfusion" form is signed (Attachment 5). In

XYZ Institution, Anywhere, USA

Institution Policy: IP-123.1
Effective Date: 1/1/96 --- Revised 3/1/96 ---
Supercedes: IP-123.1; 1/1/95
For Policy Review on: 1/1/97
Institution Applicability: _x_ Medical Center A;   _x_ Medical Center B
                                  _x_ Outpatient Surgicenter A;   _x_ HomeCare Program

addition, the physician shall write a statement in the patient's medical record reporting that the patient refused the proposed blood or blood product transfusion despite a discussion of risks and benefits and noting the patient's reasons for refusal. In this event, the Institution Risk Management Service should be consulted.

6. shall, as required by Institution Bylaws, make an entry in the progress record, at the time of discussion or as soon as possible thereafter, attesting that informed consent for blood and blood components transfusion, as defined herein, has been accomplished.

B. Autologous predonation is frequently preferable to homologous transfusion and should be encouraged when appropriate. Institutional and Local Blood Supplier policy and procedures on this option is given in the "Autologous Transfusion" document available in all Institutional Clinics (Attachment 6). This will be useful for patients to read before scheduling donations. In order to employ this option effectively;

1. the physician must assess the appropriateness of autologous blood donation for the patient, as described in "Autologous Transfusion", and must be sufficiently familiar with the patient's history and current condition to assess the safety and efficacy of autologous donation.

2. the physician must ensure the accurate completion of and must sign the "Order for Predeposit Autologous Donation" (Attachment 7) and give it to the patient.

3. the patient must make an appointment at one of the autologous donation sites available, either Institutional or Blood Supplier, as listed on the "Order for Predeposit Autologous Donation" and deliver the completed form at the time of donation.

C. Designated, Directed, or Donor-Specific Donations: State Law requires physicians to notify patients of this option. If this option is chosen, the physician must ensure the accurate completion of and must sign the "Guide for a Telephone Order for Directed Donor Blood" (Attachment 8). The physician's staff may then call the donation center to initiate a Directed Donor Blood order, and provides the donor center with the information from the completed form.

XYZ Institution, Anywhere, USA

Institution Policy: IP-123.1
Effective Date: 1/1/96 --- Revised 3/1/96 ---
Supercedes: IP-123.1; 1/1/95
For Policy Review on: 1/1/97
Institution Applicability: _x_ Medical Center A;   _x_ Medical Center B
                            _x_ Outpatient Surgicenter A;   _x_ HomeCare Program

D.   Surgery A.M. Admissions staff and Nursing Pre-op staff shall employ checklists that
     include a requirement to contact the physician if the "Transfusion Options" form is not in
     the record, if a blood type has been ordered for the patient.

E.   The adequacy of administration of Informed Consent is an ongoing Institutional Quality
     Assurance Monitor and is the responsibility of Institutional Blood Transfusion Quality
     Assurance staff. This monitor will be evaluated by the Institutional Medical Staff
     Committee Responsible for Blood Quality Assurance activity.

F.   In the event that the patient cannot sign the Consent Document due to a mechanical
     impairment in writing, or requires a surrogate decision maker, either temporarily or
     permanently, the procedure for obtaining Informed Consent for Administration of Blood
     and Blood Components must comply with the relevant provisions of the Institution
     Policy and Procedure on Informed Consent (IP-111.1) and Patient's Rights (IP-234.1).

G.   Information regarding Informed Consent for Administration of Blood and Blood
     Components will be available in the patient's Institution Medical Record and on the
     Demographics page of the Institution Computer Database. It is the responsibility of the
     physician to ensure that the Computer Database updated as necessary.

V.   Attachments:

1.   Institution Transfusion Manual for Physicians

2.   "Patient Information & Consent - Transfusion Options and Alternatives"; Institution
     Form 123-456

3.   "A Patient's Guide to Blood Transfusion"

4.   "Institution Universal Consent to Invasive Procedure"

5.   "Refusal to Permit Blood Transfusion"

6.   Joint Institution & Blood Supplier Policy; "Autologous Transfusion"

XYZ Institution, Anywhere, USA

Institution Policy: IP-123.1
Effective Date: 1/1/96 --- Revised 3/1/96 ---
Supercedes: IP-123.1; 1/1/95
For Policy Review on: 1/1/97
Institution Applicability: _x_ Medical Center A;   _x_ Medical Center B
                                _x_ Outpatient Surgicenter A;   _x_ HomeCare Program

7. "Order for Predeposit Autologous Donation"

8. "Guide for a Telephone Order for Directed Donor Blood"

Appendix 7-2. Example of Informed Consent for Transfusion Included in a General Informed Consent Policy

HOSPITAL POLICY MANUAL

Policy Title: Informed Consent

Approval By: Medical Policy Committee·

Approval Date: 03/06/94

Effective Date: 04/01/94

Replaces: Informed Consent, version 10/01/91

A.   Purpose

A physician performing a medical or surgical procedure on a patient must obtain the patient's informed consent to the procedure. This is essential to medical practice. It is also required by law.

B.   Elements of Informed Consent

Informed consent involves a process of effective communication in which the physician must provide adequate information for the patient to make an informed judgement on the proposed treatment. Specifically, the physician must disclose in a reasonable manner all significant medical information that a) the physician possesses or reasonably should possess as a physician with appropriate knowledge and technical skill practicing in that specialty, and b) is material to an intelligent decision by the patient. Information is material to the patient's decision if a reasonable person in the patient's position would consider it a significant factor in deciding whether or not to undergo the procedure. This information should include:

1.   The nature of the patient's condition;

2.   The proposed treatment and possible alternatives (including no treatment);

3.   The benefits of the proposed treatment and alternatives;

4.   The nature and probability of risks of the proposed

treatment and alternatives;

5.   The inability of the physician to predict results and the irreversibility of the procedure, when that is the case;

6.   The role (if any) played by residents, fellows, and students in medical and allied disciplines in providing the proposed treatment; and

7.   The possible use in education and research of blood or tissue removed from the patient and not needed for further medical care.

The information which must be provided will vary according to the patient's intelligence, experience, age and other similar factors.   Information the physician reasonably believes is already known to the patient need not be specifically disclosed.

C.   <u>Applicability of Informed Consent Policy</u>

Under hospital policy, the physician must document, on the approved hospital form, consent for all therapeutic and diagnostic procedures where disclosure of significant medical information, including major risks involved, would assist a patient in making an informed decision whether to undergo the proposed procedure.   Such procedures include but are not limited to:

a.   Transfusion of blood components
b.   etc.

Exceptions:

1.   Emergencies: A procedure on the above list may be performed without obtaining consent in advance in an emergency when the patient's wellbeing would seriously be endangered by withholding treatment until consent can be obtained.

2.   Patient is physically incapable or mentally incompetent to sign a consent form

2

      a.   (Describe suitable alternative procedures including use of guardian and surrogates.)

   3.   Minors - If the patient is under eighteen years of age, consent should be obtained and documented in the otherwise usual manner from the patient's parents. Consent by a minor without parental consent is legally appropriate in the care of:

(Discussion of care of minors, emancipated minors and mature minors)

D.   <u>Frequency of Informed Consent</u>

Informed consent shall be obtained before each event listed in C, above. Patients in certain therapeutic programs listed below involving multiple treatments (inpatient, outpatient, or mixed) may consent to an entire course of routine therapy prior to the first treatment, and a single consent form may be signed for the entire course of treatment, if:

1.   The entire course of treatment is disclosed, consented to, and documented;

2.   No material change occurs in:

    a.   the risks and benefits;
    b.   the mode of treatment; or
    c.   the patient's competence to consent; and

3.   Consent is re-obtained and re-documented at least annually.

Therapeutic programs covered by this exception include but are not limited to the following:

    a.   Repetitive red blood cell or platelet transfusions to patients with marrow aplasia during a single admission;
    b.   Peritoneal dialysis and hemodialysis;
    c.   Series of plasmapheresis procedures;
    d.

E.   Responsible Personnel

Informed consent shall be obtained by a physician. The best
practice is for the physician performing or supervising the
procedure to obtain and document the informed consent.   On
resident services, a resident with primary responsibility for
the patient who will be performing or supervising the
procedure would generally be the appropriate person to obtain
consent. The physician who obtains the consent should explain
that other personnel, including residents, fellows, and
students in medical and allied disciplines may participate in
the procedure. The consent may be obtained and the form may
be completed in an physician's office but, if so, the form
must nevertheless be placed in the hospital record, in
approximate chronological order, prior to the preparation of
the patient for the procedure.

F.   Documentation

The standard hospital forms, copies of which are appended to
this policy, must be used for documenting consent in any case
involving a procedure for which documented consent is required
under this policy.   While physicians are encouraged to
supplement the information on the standard form, none of the
information on the form shall be deleted. If documentation on
a form is not required, it is nevertheless highly desirable to
write a note in the chart indicating that consent has been
obtained.   In the case of procedures for which documented
consent is not required, a clinical unit may at its discretion
develop and use special consent forms. Where a different form
is required by law or other hospital policy, consent must be
documented on that form.

G.   Monitoring for Compliance

The Hospital's Medical Policy Committee is charged with
overseeing compliance with this policy and recommending
further guidelines as indicated.   The Quality Assurance
Committee will institute procedures for screening records to
insure that informed consent has been documented in the manner
provided by this policy and will regularly bring compliance
data for individual departments and services to the Medical
Policy Committee.

4

Appendix 7-3. Example of a Separate Procedure for Informed Consent for Transfusion

INSTITUTION NAME

POLICY AND PROCEDURE MANUAL

SUBJECT:	Section: Patient Care	No. of Pages: 2
Transfusion Informed Consent	Index Under: Transfusion of Blood Components	Effective Date:
Supersedes:		Scope: Medical Center

1.0 Policy:

    1.1 All patients will be given information concerning the transfusion of blood components prior to administration. A Transfusion Informed Consent form will be completed by the physician and booklet given to the patient prior to the transfusion of blood components.

    1.2 This form shall be completed for each surgical procedure or prior to the treatment plan for a specific diagnosis (i.e., completed courses of chemotherapy of bone marrow transplantation "BMT"). EXCEPTION: A patient undergoing right atrial catheter (RAC) for BMT or RAC for chemotherapy does not need a second transfusion form signed. The signed form will be kept in the Transfusion Medicine Section of the Medical Record or there will be evidence on the face sheet that a form has been signed previously.

2.0 Procedure - Inpatient:

    2.1 The RN/LVN will initiate the transfusion when there is a completed form or evidence on the face sheet that a form has been signed previously. If a form is not in place or evidence of previously signed form is not found, the nurse will notify the physician prior to any transfusion.

        2.1.1 The signed Transfusion Informed Consent will be given to the nurse.

        2.1.2 The completed form will be placed in the Transfusion Medicine section of the Medical Record.

        2.1.3 Using the CareNet System, the nurse or clerk will send the Admitting Department the message "Transfusion Information signed", the date and his/her name.

        2.1.4 The Admitting Department will receive this information and produce a new Inpatient/Outpatient Admission form (face sheet).

Institution Name

```
┌─────────────────────┐
│ Transfusion Informed │
│ Consent              │
└─────────────────────┘
```

2.1.5   The new face sheet will be delivered to the Inpatient/Outpatient departments by the Admitting staff the following day.

2.1.6   The nursing clerk will place the new Inpatient/Outpatient Admission form in the Progress Notes Section of the Medical Record.

2.1.7   Upon discharge, the Inpatient/Outpatient Admission form will be placed on the front of the medical record.

3.0   Procedure - Outpatient:

3.1   The RN/LVN will check the medical record for a signed transfusion form or will notify the physician to have one signed.

3.2   The nurse, after checking what date the consent was signed will write that date on the face sheet in the outpatient record. He/she will record "Transfusion Informed Consent signed", the date and his/her name.

3.3   A log will be kept in each clinic area which will show those patients who have signed the Transfusion Informed Consent. This log will contain the patient's name, chart number and the date.

3.4   The new entries in the log will be given to the Admitting Department on a daily basis. The information will be taken from the log and put into the computer system by the Admitting Personnel, but a new face sheet for outpatients will not be generated. This will make the information available for the inpatient wings should the patient be admitted but new paperwork will not be generated for filing in the Medical Record Department.

3.5   For any outpatient who signs a Transfusion Informed Consent and is admitted the same day, the Admitting Staff will carry to the patient wings, the new outpatient face sheet as well as the new inpatient face sheet. The outpatient face sheet will be placed behind the new inpatient face sheet in the Inpatient Medical Record.

INFORMED CONSENT FOR BLOOD TRANSFUSION: PHYSICIAN'S CHECKLIST

Patient Name: _____   Record No. _____
Diagnosis: _____   Date: _____
Type of Procedure: _____   Date: _____

_____ Is there a reasonable possibility that a blood/component transfusion will be required?
      _____ Red Blood Cells
      _____ FFP
      _____ Platelets
      _____ Cryo or fibrin sealant
      _____ Clotting Concentrate
      _____ IVIG

Have relevant transfusion alternatives been considered?
      _____ DDAVP, Aprotinin, EACA, Vitamin K

Is there an indication for a special component:
      _____ CMV safe
      _____ Leukocyte-reduced
      _____ Irradiated

_____ Will the patient benefit from Autologous blood?
      _____ If yes, is the patient a candidate for autologous donation?
      _____ Estimate the number of units desired.
      _____ Arrangements made for units to be drawn?

_____ Does the patient wish to have Donor Specific Donations?
      _____ If yes, have arrangements been made for donors to be screened?

_____ Is intra- or post-operative salvage a reasonable consideration?

_____ Has the procedure and the possibility of blood use been discussed with the patient?
      _____ If yes, has the patient been informed of the reasonable risks of blood transfusion?
      _____ Has the patient been given relevant educational materials?
      _____ Has the patient had ample opportunity to ask questions?
      _____ Does the patient understand all relevant transfusion options?
            (Autologous, Donor Specific, Salvage)

_____ Has a consent form been signed and/or note written in chart?

_____ Has relevant information been conveyed to other key members of the health care team?
      Family, Nurses, Operating Room, Transfusion Service, Blood Bank, Home Care

Informed Consent for Blood Transfusion: Nurse's Checklist

Patient Name: _____   Record No. _____

Diagnosis: _____   Date: _____

Type of Procedure: _____   Date: _____

_____ Is the consent form present in the medical chart or note written by the physician?

_____ If yes, is the consent form signed and dated?

_____ If no, is there evidence on the face sheet that a form had been signed previously?

_____ Is there a need to obtain a renewed new consent form?

_____ If yes, has the patient's physician been notified to obtain a consent?

INFORMED CONSENT FOR TRANSFUSION FORM
(Paul Gann Blood Safety Act, Health & Safety Code S 1645)

INSTRUCTIONS: PLEASE SELECT <u>ONLY</u> ONE

PatientName _____

1. I have provided the patient with the State Department of Health Services standardized written summary concerning the advantages, disadvantages, risks and benefits of autologous blood and of directed and nondirected homologous blood from volunteers ("DHS Pamphlet"). I have also allowed adequate time prior to the patient's medical or surgical procedure(s) for the patient to arrange for a directed donation or for the patient to donate his/her own blood.

                                     Physician's
Date: _____   Signature: _____

Received by: _____ Date: _____
                   (Patient's Signature)

2. I have provided the patient with the DHS pamphlet, however, the patient has voluntarily waived his/her right of pre-donation or is ineligible to donate because of pre-existing medical condition(s).

                                     Physician's
Date: _____   Signature: _____

Received by: _____ Date: _____
                   (Patient's Signature)

3. Because I have determined that there is not a reasonable possibility that a blood transfusion may be necessary as a result of the medical or surgical procedure(s) the patient will undergo, I have <u>not</u> provided the patient with the DHS pamphlet.

                                     Physician's
Date: _____   Signature: _____

4. Because of life-threatening emergencyor medical contraindication(s), I have <u>not</u> provided the patient with the DHS pamphlet and I have not allowed time prior to the patient's medical or surgical procedure(s) for pre-donation to occur.

                                     Physician's
Date: _____   Signature: _____

City of Hope National Medical Center   **ADDRESSOGRAPH:**
TRANSFUSION INFORMATION FORM
(Paul Gann Blood Safety Act,
Health & Safety Code S1645)

The Safest Blood is Your Own.
Use It Whenever Possible.

Many surgeries do not require blood transfusions. However, if you need blood, you have several options. Although you have the right to refuse a blood transfusion, this decision may hold life-threatening consequences. Please carefully review this brochure and decide with your doctor which option(s) you prefer.

PLEASE NOTE: Your options may be limited by time and health factors, so it is important to begin carrying out your decision as soon as possible.

A Patient's Guide to Blood Transfusions

- ASK YOUR PHYSICIAN ABOUT NEW DEVELOPMENTS IN TRANSFUSION MEDICINE.
- CHECK WITH YOUR INSURANCE COMPANY FOR THEIR REIMBURSEMENT POLICY.

This brochure was developed by
California Department of Health Services
714/744 P Street
Sacramento, CA 95814
Kenneth W. Kizer, M.D., M.P.H., Director

This brochure is distributed by
Medical Board of California
1426 Howe Avenue
Sacramento, CA 95825-3236
Kenneth J. Wagstaff, Executive Director

ORDER ADDITIONAL COPIES BY SENDING A CHECK OR
MONEY ORDER TO "STATE OF CALIFORNIA" TO:

Department of General Services
Office of Procurement, Publications Section
P.O. Box 1015
North Highlands, CA 95660

Ask for "IF YOU NEED BLOOD" sold in bundles of 50 copies
at $ 10.00 per bundle. Cost is likely to increase in 1991.
(NOTE: This publication is not copyrighted. You may
duplicate for distribution to your patients.)

If You Need Blood...

The methods of using your own blood can be used independently or together to eliminate or minimize the need for donor blood, as well as virtually eliminate transfusion risks of infection and allergic reaction.

■ AUTOLOGOUS BLOOD - Using Your Own Blood

Option	Explanation	Advantages	Disadvantages
PRE-OPERATIVE DONATION Donating Your Own Blood Before Surgery	The blood bank draws your blood and stores it until you need it, during or after surgery. For elective surgery only.	✓ Eliminates or minimizes the need for someone else's blood during and after surgery.	• Requires advance planning • May delay surgery. • Medical conditions may prevent pre-operative donation.
INTRA-OPERATIVE AUTOLOGOUS TRANSFUSION Recycling Your Blood During Surgery	Instead of being discarded, blood lost during surgery is filtered, and put back into your body during surgery. For elective and emergency surgery.	✓ Eliminates or minimizes need for someone else's blood during surgery. Large amounts of blood can be recycled.	• Not for use if cancer or infection is present.
POST-OPERATIVE AUTOLOGOUS TRANSFUSION Recycling Your Blood After Surgery	Blood lost after surgery is collected, filtered and returned. For elective and emergency surgery.	✓ Eliminates or minimizes the need for someone else's blood after surgery.	• Not for use if cancer or infection is present.
HEMODILUTION Donating Your Own Blood During Surgery	Immediately before surgery, some of your blood is taken and replaced with I.V. fluids. After surgery, your blood is filtered and returned to you. For elective surgery.	✓ Eliminates or minimizes the need for someone else's blood during and after surgery. Dilutes your blood so you lose less concentrated blood during surgery.	• Limited number of units can be drawn. • Medical conditions may prevent hemodilution.
APHERESIS Donating Your Own Platelets and Plasma	Before surgery, your platelets and plasma, which help stop bleeding, are withdrawn, filtered, and returned to you when you need it. For elective surgery.	✓ May eliminate the need for donor platelets and plasma, especially in high blood-loss procedures.	• Medical conditions may prevent apheresis. • Procedure has limited application.

In some cases, you may require more blood than anticipated. If this happens and you receive blood other than your own, there is a possibility of complications, such as hepatitis or AIDS.

■ DONOR BLOOD - Using Someone Else's Blood

Donor blood and blood products can never be absolutely 100% safe, even though testing makes the risk very small.

Option	Explanation	Advantages	Disadvantages
VOLUNTEER BLOOD From the Community Blood Supply	Blood and blood products donated by volunteer donors to a community blood bank.	✓ Readily available. Can be life-saving when your own blood is not available.	• Risk of disease transmission (such as hepatitis or AIDS), and allergic reactions.
Note: You may wish to check whether donors are paid or volunteer, since blood from commercial (paid) donors may not, in some cases, be as safe as blood from volunteers.			
DESIGNATED DONOR BLOOD From Donors You Select	Blood and blood donors you select who must meet the same requirements as volunteer donors.	✓ You can select people with your own blood type who you feel are safe donors.	• Risk of disease transmission (such as hepatitis or AIDS), and allergic reactions. • May require several days of advanced donation. • Not necessarily as safe, nor safer, than volunteer donor blood.
Note: Care should be taken in selecting donors. Donors should never be pressured into donating. Donations from certain family members may require irradiation of blood.			

FORM NO. 7067-C007

81 62440

Appendix 7-4. Example of Informed Consent for Transfusion Included in a Transfusion Procedure

STANDARD OPERATING PROCEDURE

TITLE: Administration of Whole Blood, Packed Red Blood Cells, Saline Washed Red Cells, Frozen Deglycerolized Red Cells

Effective Date: Approved By:

Replaces: Approval Date:

Level of Personnel: Qualified RNs

Designated Clinical Area: All

Applicable Policy Statements:

Written informed consent must be obtained from patients prior to transfusion of blood, its components, or blood derivatives.

Blood transfusions are initiated only upon a written order by a licensed physician. The order should include the date, name of the component, amount, and if possible, rate of infusion.   Orders should be written on the day of transfusions.   Transfusions not given on the day ordered may be carried over one day.   Standing orders for blood and blood components are unacceptable.

Blood and its components or derivatives should be administered through a separate administration set. Never infuse blood and IV fluids simultaneously through the same site.

Equipment

Red cell component
Blood recipient set with 170 micron filter
19 gauge 1" needle
Alcohol prep pad
Tape
(Equipment for inserting IV if patient does not have one)

Nursing Actions:

1.   Confirm that order is written by physician.

2.   Confirm that patient has signed a transfusion consent form.
     If consent has not been signed, page patient's physician and
     inform of need for consent.

3.   Make positive patient identification by (describe procedure).

4.   Verify that the unit of blood is the correct unit for the
     patient by (describe two person check system).

5.   Verify that the blood component and the recipient are ABO and
     Rh compatible by (describe procedure).

6.   Inspect the unit of blood for discoloration, air bubbles and
     grossly visible clots. Return unit to blood bank if the unit
     appears to be unsuitable (describe).

7   Set up the equipment for transfusion (at bedside). Open one
     tab port of the bag and insert the blood recipient set into
     this port. Close clamp of administration set.

(8. Describe remainder of procedure.)

Documentation

Record date, time transfusion was initiated and completed, and
signature on blood requisition which accompanies the blood
component and place in miscellaneous section of patient's record.

Record two person verification of patient and blood unit identity
on the blood requisition in the appropriate space.

Record patient vital signs on flow sheet.

References

Vengelen-Tyler V, ed. Technical manual, 12th ed. Bethesda,
MD: American Association of Blood Banks, 1996.

Hospital Policy Manual

2

Appendix 7-5. Association Bulletin #94-3. Informed Consent for Blood Transfusion

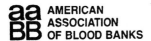 AMERICAN
ASSOCIATION
OF BLOOD BANKS

ASSOCIATION BULLETIN

94-3

DATE: September 1, 1994

TO: AABB Institutional Members

FROM: Charles H. Wallas, MD   Jo Ann Hoffman
          President   Acting Chief Executive Officer

RE: Informed Consent for Blood Transfusion

The AABB Board of Directors has revised and reaffirmed the Association's position on informed consent for blood transfusion, and a copy is provided for your information.

This will be included in a 1995 edition of the AABB publication, *Informed Consent for Blood Transfusion: A Physicians Resource Kit*, which is in the process of being updated and expanded by the AABB Scientific Section Coordinating Committee. The 1989 *Kit* has become outdated and used alone may no longer provide adequate or accurate information for obtaining informed consent. In particular, continued showing of the video to patients and/or use of the information sheets without supplemental, updated information is discouraged.

This Association Bulletin supersedes the July 10, 1986, AABB memorandum to institutional members, *Informed Consent for Blood Transfusion.*

Informed Consent for Blood Transfusion

The AABB recommends that patients who receive non-emergent transfusions be informed of the risks and benefits of blood and blood components and consent to their use.

<u>Elements of Informed Consent</u>

The general elements for informed consent include:

1)   an understanding of what medical action is recommended;
2)   its associated risks and benefits;
3)   alternative methods of therapy available and their attendant risks including the possible consequences of not receiving the recommended therapy;
4)   an opportunity to ask questions; and
5)   consent to transfusion.

The Blood Bank and/or Medical Director of the Blood Bank can provide important information to treating physicians about transfusion therapy and may participate in the development of informed consent policies. The AABB does not, however, advise that the Blood Bank and/or Medical Director of the Blood Bank be the instrument of implementation, enforcement or monitoring of informed consent, which are the responsibilities of the treating physician.

<u>Documentation</u>

The most important part of this process is communication between doctor and patient. It is essential that this communication be documented. This documentation may be accomplished in several ways. The following methods of documentation have been considered appropriate:

1)   A written progress note in the patient's medical record which includes elements of the process of informed consent; or

2)   An informed consent form.

A single informed consent may be sufficient for any course of therapy which may include one or more transfusions, during one or more treatment episodes.

<u>State Law</u>

State law may dictate required elements of informed consent for transfusion, and should be consulted.

Adopted 7/10/86, Revised 7/28/94

Index